Medieval Communities and the Mad

Medieval Communities and the Mad

Narratives of Crime and Mental Illness in Late Medieval France

Aleksandra Pfau

Routledge
Taylor & Francis Group
LONDON AND NEW YORK

First published in 2021 by Amsterdam University Press Ltd.

Published 2025 by Routledge
4 Park Square, Milton Park, Abingdon, Oxon OX14 4RN
605 Third Avenue, New York, NY 10158

Routledge is an imprint of the Taylor & Francis Group, an informa business

ISBN: 9789462983359 (hbk)
ISBN: 9781041182696 (pbk)
ISBN: 9781003699576 (ebk)
NUR 613

Cover illustration: Mort de Léarchos from a fifteenth-century manuscript of Laurent de Premierfait's *Des Cas des Nobles Hommes et Femmes*
Source: Bibliothèque nationale de France français 229 folio 11

Cover design: Coördesign, Leiden

DOI: 10.5117/9789462983359

For Product Safety Concerns and Information please contact our EU representative:
GPSR@taylorandfrancis.com
Taylor & Francis Verlag GmbH, Kaufingerstraße 24, 80331 München, Germany

Table of Contents

List of Tables

Acknowledgments

I would like to thank my colleagues at Hendrix College for their generous support of my continuing research for this book project. I am also grateful for the staff of the Archives Nationales microfilm room. The research began during my graduate work at the University of Michigan, and it was shaped in important ways by the guidance of Helmut Puff, Diane Owen Hughes, Peggy McCracken, and Michael MacDonald. However, it would never have come to fruition without the support and occasional prodding of my mentor, Wendy Turner. I would also like to thank the anonymous reviewers and the editorial board who provided excellent suggestions for how to improve the work. There are too many other individuals who have contributed to this project in large and small ways while I have worked on it over the last fifteen years for me to thank them all here, but I will be eternally grateful for all the conversations that helped me refine and reshape my ideas. Finally, all my love to David and Rachel, who lived with this project for many years.

Introduction

Abstract
The concept of madness as a challenge to communities lies at the core of legal sources. This book considers how communal networks, ranging from the locale to the realm, responded to people who were considered mad. The madness of individuals played a role in engaging communities with legal mechanisms and proto-national identity constructs, as petitioners sought the king's mercy as an alternative to local justice. The resulting narratives about the mentally ill in late medieval France constructed madness as an inability to live according to communal rules. Although such texts defined madness through acts that threatened social bonds, those ties were reaffirmed through the medium of the remission letter. The composers of the letters presented madness as a communal concern, situating the mad within the household, where care could be provided. These mad were usually not expelled but integrated, often through pilgrimage, surveillance, or chains, into their kin and communal relationships.

Keyterms: Madness, Insanity Defense, Pardon, Community

In August of 1350, the first Valois King of France, Philip VI, granted a pardon to one Jehan le Vignon. As his children explained, Jehan had been 'out of his senses and all good memory' for the past three years, such that he had tried to kill himself by throwing himself into a well. It was only through the 'diligence' of his wife Richeu and his four children, Jencon, Marie, Jehanne, and Ysabeau that he was not able to commit suicide. However, the Thursday after the feast of Saint James in July their attention wavered enough that Jehan was able to pick up a stick and hit his wife on the back of the head. Their children noted that she may have died partly from her 'frailty and ancient age of seventy-two years or thereabouts'. Regardless, Jehan was taken up by the local officers of justice, and his children feared that he might be put to death. Thus, they brought the case to the king's attention, requesting that he pardon their father and allow him to return to the family's care.

Pfau, A., *Medieval Communities and the Mad: Narratives of Crime and Mental Illness in Late Medieval France*. Taylor & Francis Group, 2021
DOI: 10.5117/9789462983359_INTRO

Philip agreed, on condition that in future Jehan must stay 'in the care of the above said supplicants, his children'.[1]

Madness has often been imagined as an isolating condition, in terms of both the nature of the condition itself and the way the mentally ill have historically been treated. The kinds of intellectual histories that have been written about insanity in the Middle Ages tend to support this view, focusing on theoretical treatises and literary treatments of the mad.[2] More recent work has shifted to consider the wider social significance of the disease, acknowledging that madness is a social condition and examining the ways that families and communities coped with individuals they identified as mad.[3] Jehan le Vignon was clearly not an isolated figure, abandoned by his family or his community. Rather, his wife and children banded together to ensure that he was unable to harm himself, and when, despite their efforts, he harmed his wife, his children fought to have him released from prison and returned to their care. This book examines Jehan le Vignon and others whose stories appear in the collection of pardons granted by the king of France. Historians have suggested that medieval concepts of social identity were defined through membership in multiple communities.[4] Thus, the communities examined in this book range from the vastness of Christendom as a whole and the French realm, down to local villages and particular kin groups. Rather than being marginalized, mad people became central to narratives which sought to ameliorate the damage they had done and begin the process of reconstructing their fractured communities, not by isolating or imprisoning them, but by ensuring familial or communal care. However, it is important to note that community is not always supportive, and family or communal care was not always easy or successful. Embedded within the narrative about Jehan le Vignon's crime, we can see the fissures and failures of care in the community. In restructuring the community around the very individual whose actions threaten it, these letters reimagine and reform communal participation and belonging.

1 Archives Nationales Series JJ book 78, folio 145, recto number 262 (henceforth abbreviated as AN JJ 78 fo 145 no 262; verso folios will be indicated with a v): 'hors de son sens et de tout bon memoir'; 'diligence'; 'sa frelesse et ancienete de laage de soixante douze ans ou environ'; 'en la garde des dessus dis supplians ses enfans'. Transcriptions and translations are mine unless otherwise indicated.

2 See particularly Huot 2003, Fritz 1992, Laharie 1991, Neaman 1975, and Doob 1974.

3 For the most important recent work in this area, see Ternon 2018, Ternon 2015, Mellyn 2014, Trenery 2019, and Turner 2013a.

4 Bynum 1984, pp. 82–109; Watt 1997, pp. 1–19.

I. Language and Narrative

Following in the footsteps of scholars including Erik Midelfort and Elizabeth Mellyn, I have chosen to use madness as an overarching term in this book in an effort to access broader linguistic, social, cultural, and political meanings.[5] The French language in the Middle Ages had a multiplicity of terms and phrases to describe the elusive condition of mental disturbance. Indeed, as a condition that was recognized through behavioral patterns, that was described in terms of a rupture of communal expectations, and that infringed upon many social concerns, madness was peculiarly suited to linguistic exchange. The languages of the law, of medicine, of religion, and of literature each borrowed extensively from one another in efforts to depict the state of madness. Many texts use descriptive phrases, such as the French phrase *hors de son sens* ('out of their senses') rather than just one word, as we still do in modern discourse when we refer to people who are 'out of their minds' or who 'come back to their senses'. Modern terminology includes some of the same range of possibilities as medieval terminology, and the large scope of the term 'madness' allows for this expanse. 'Madness' also avoids enforcing modern anachronistic understandings that were not always present in the vast array of terms used in medieval texts to describe this condition. Insanity insists on an interpretation that pairs madness as the opposite of sanity, or health, and mental illness is equally focused on diseases of the mind. While both of these concepts existed in the Middle Ages, there were also a number of alternative ways of thinking about what madness was and what it meant, as there are now. The ideas of 'not sane', 'foolish', 'mentally ill', and 'mentally disturbed' do have their place within the greater conceptualization of madness. Therefore, I will use all these terms according to context, with 'madness' as an umbrella under which the others can be found. The term madness, rather than limiting my focus to a single lens, allows the engagement of a range of interpretive frameworks.

In using a term that allows for a large array of discourses, I am also conscious of the narrative nature of my sources. This book focuses on French letters of remission as the main source base because of the richness of the narratives contained within these texts. Pardons originated in the early fourteenth century, when the French king began to demonstrate his grace

5 Midelfort 1999, pp. 11; Mellyn 2014, p. 19. I acknowledge that this is a fraught term, as the work by disability activists and the recent 'Mad Studies' movement demonstrate. See Beresford 2019. Nevertheless, because I am writing about people who were labeled by their contemporaries, I find it a useful term of analysis.

and mercy by granting remission for crimes. The criminal, or the criminal's family members, with the help of a royal notary, told the story of the crime, focusing on the details of the event and providing background information as the narrator deemed appropriate. Remission was only available for crimes for which the punishment was death, and the pardon rhetorically erased the crime, not only on the level of government officials, who could no longer pursue the pardoned criminal for that crime, but also on the level of the community, since the letter restored the criminal to his or her 'good reputation and renown'. 'Good reputation', as Ron Akehurst has argued, was a legal category that could affect a person and his or her family's standing in civil cases, ability to make contracts, and likelihood of conviction in criminal cases.[6] At the same time, as Barbara Hanawalt has shown, 'good reputation' was also a social category, determined by and affecting one's standing in the community,[7] and threats to an individual's reputation could threaten the reputation of the entire family. Of course, despite the rhetorical claim that remission letters erased the crime, many of the acts that were pardoned in these letters could never truly be undone. Jehan le Vignon's wife could not be brought back to life, and his family could not be fully restored. While all remission letters were intended to erase the crime and to represent it as an aberration in an otherwise good lifestyle, the small fraction of letters that used the language of madness sought to remove the crime even more fully from the identity of the perpetrator, since medieval law asserted that the mad lacked intent for their actions.[8] At the same time, however, deploying the language of madness could be a risk for the composers of the letter, since the reading of a remission letter was a public act and admission of madness could have longer-term repercussions. As a result, the choice to craft a narrative of madness was not a common one.

Through the letter of remission, the French king was making a number of claims about his personal authority. At the same time, however, as the largest output of the French royal chancery from the 1350s, remission letters also demonstrated the ability of the French bureaucracy to continue to function through instability and conquest. Increasingly throughout the

6 Akehurst 2003.

7 Hanawalt 1998, esp. pp. 1–4.

8 Despite Guido Ruggiero's assertion that Venice in the early Renaissance was unusual in refusing to hold mad people responsible for crimes because it was ruled by bankers and merchants who were more practical (1982), this practice originates in Roman law and was commonly recognized everywhere in the Middle Ages. In general, see Walker 1985. For France, see Fritz 1992, pp. 153–164. For England, see Green 1972. For Florence, see Mellyn 2014, pp. 58–93. For Germany, see Midelfort 1999, pp. 187–196.

late-fourteenth and early-fifteenth centuries, the individual holding the French crown was unable to personally engage with the petitions of his subjects, yet the language of the remission letters obscured these truths. Through the letter, the French king was likened to God, whose powers of grace and mercy allowed him to act above the law. From the perspective of supplicants, this meant that the remission letters did not need to follow a prescribed storyline to ensure validation.[9] Nevertheless, some mutually agreed version of 'truth' was necessary, since the letter had to be read aloud by the local judge in the presence of the adverse party, and if they raised an objection the remission could be annulled. Remission letters were also expensive, and to get them ratified a petitioner had to travel to the king's council, which could be difficult, particularly for people who did not live in or around Paris. The price was officially set at 32 sous in the fourteenth century, more than a week's wages for most artisans, and each step had charges attached to it, so the final price could be much higher.[10] Access to such letters, then, often required assistance from family or friends. In cases of mad perpetrators, like Jehan le Vignon, remission was only possible through the intervention of his relatives, specifically his children, who asked the king to pardon their father for killing their mother. Despite the ways that Jehan le Vignon's crime tore at the very fabric of the family, his children sought a pardon, promising to care for him in their household rather than allowing him to face justice for his crime.

Since the 1980s, the 'linguistic turn' in history writing has made historians more conscious of how language shapes the writing of history in multiple and complex ways.[11] Historians have been reminded that their documents, as well as their own historical narratives, have been shaped by discourse, narrative, and literary conventions. Subsequently, the profession has become more critical of the ability of texts to reflect what actually happened in the past. As John Toews claims in a 1987 review essay, at the very least historians

> seem ready to concede that language can no longer be construed as simply a medium, relatively or potentially transparent, for the representation or expression of a reality outside of itself and are willing to entertain seriously some form of semiological theory in which language is conceived

9 As distinct from the English law courts, where there were strict conditions for proving madness, which caused a certain amount of conformity among cases. See Green 1972, p. 680.

10 Gauvard 1991, v. I, p. 68.

11 The phrase 'linguistic turn' was first used in the title of a collection of essays in 1967; see Rorty.

> of as a self-contained system of 'signs' whose meanings are determined by their relations to each other, rather than by their relation to some 'transcendental' or extralinguistic object or subject.[12]

This focus on semiotics was part of a movement towards interdisciplinarity, or at least towards mining other disciplines, including philosophy, literary studies, and cultural anthropology, for useful theoretical tools. For example, in 1981, Natalie Zemon Davis pointed out the increasing use of the works of anthropologists such as Mary Douglas, E. E. Evans-Pritchard, Clifford Geertz, and Victor Turner, especially among medieval and early modern historians who were seeking a way to comprehend events that had previously 'been defined by historians as irrational or superstitious, or as an arbitrary cover for real and serious social and political conflicts'. Where historians attempted to dismiss descriptions of such events as spirit possession and witchcraft accusations, anthropologists 'have such events at the center of their observation'.[13] Anthropological works have thus allowed historians to take certain phenomena or descriptions seriously, considering the meanings that contemporaries saw in these events.

Davis also stressed the relevance of literary theory in her 1987 book on remission letters (or pardon tales), provocatively entitled *Fiction in the Archives*. She encouraged historians to confront the particular way that their sources are informed by narrative construction. Her focus is on the 'fictional' aspects of the documents, by which she explains she 'do[es] not mean their feigned elements, but rather, using the other and broader sense of the root word *fingere*, their forming, shaping, and molding elements: the crafting of a narrative'.[14] This awareness of and, more significantly, valuation of narrative provides much richer analytical possibilities than the discarding of narrative elements in search of a hidden 'truth' common in historicist practice. Davis reveals the ways 'information, values, and language habits could flow across lines of class and culture', arguing that supplicants, listeners, and pardoners 'were all implicated in a common discourse about violence and its pacification'.[15] Her project provides a model for thinking about narratives like those addressed in this book. How were stories about madness and crime constructed, and what distinguishes them from other narratives?

12 Toews 1987, pp. 881–882.
13 Davis 1981, p. 268.
14 Davis 1987, p. 3.
15 Davis 1987, p. 112.

In the 1990s, gender historians above all took on the challenge of thinking through the implications of linguistic concerns for history as a discipline, in particular the suggestion that language 'not only shapes experienced reality but constitutes it'.[16] In what has emerged as a classical formulation, Joan Scott's 1991 essay argues that historians 'need to attend to the historical processes that, through discourse, position subjects and produce their experiences. It is not individuals who have experience, but subjects who are constituted through experience'.[17] As Gabrielle Spiegel notes in her introduction to a 2005 reprinting of Scott's essay, however, many historians prefer 'to see language as the place where experience is made meaningful via a creative appropriation of the conditions of daily life, rather than created'.[18]

Indeed, in her own work, Spiegel has grappled with the relationship between language and experience, proposing a 'middle ground' that attempts to mediate between acknowledging the importance of language and discourse and the historians' desire for empirical research.[19] She posited in 1997 that

> the power and the meaning of any given set of representations derive in large part from their social context and their relation to the social and political networks in which they are elaborated. Even if one accepts the poststructuralist argument that language constitutes the social world of meaning, it is possible to maintain that language itself acquires meaning and authority only within specific social and historical settings.[20]

This need to examine what Spiegel calls the 'social logic of the text' rests on a recognition of language as constituted as well as constitutive. It focuses attention not only on how texts are discursively inscribed but also on how they are embedded within particular social contexts. This interest in language and discourse is particularly useful for discussions of madness, in part because mad historical actors so seldom speak for themselves. In

16 Toews 1987, p. 882. Many historians have been troubled by the implications of this theory, objecting to the more radical interpretations that deny any reality in the past. See Richard Evans 1999.

17 Scott 2005, p. 203. In her critical response, Kathleen Canning contends that Scott ignores the mutually constitutive nature of experience and language. Canning posits that the key to 'analyzing how discourses change, how subjects contest power in its discursive form, and how their desires and discontents transform or explode discursive systems is the concept of agency'. Canning 2006, p. 76.

18 Spiegel 2005, p. 200.

19 Spiegel 1997, pp. 44–56.

20 Spiegel 1997, p. 53.

facing the aftermath of a crime committed by a mad person, people came to terms with madness as a social, not just individual, phenomenon.

The impetus to consider the linguistic and narrative nature of the texts that historians use equally opens into questions about historical narratives as shaped and constructed by historians.[21] What role does the historian now play in relation to her documents? John Arnold, in his work on the Inquisition in southern France, responds to this question by challenging the historian's 'desire to establish whether or not we can "trust" the sources'.[22] He suggests that the power relationships that led to the creation of these particular documents be brought to the fore, not to deconstruct them and reveal the underlying 'truths', but rather for what these power relationships can tell us about themselves.[23] Cordelia Beattie, who uses legal documents to talk about the lives of women, also refuses to discard the structures that brought these documents into being. She notes that 'the petition and the answer do not allow access to unmediated voices, that the structure and language of the petition and the answer were affected by the involvement of lawyers and the nature of the court' and suggests that 'recognition of the limitations of the evidence is not to give up on historical subjects but rather a refusal to simplify their lives, which were lived within discursive systems'.[24] As Sarah Maza notes in her discussion of crime narratives in pre-Revolutionary France, '[s]tories give us both an individual and a collective sense of identity and purpose; they can undermine our world just as easily as they order and confirm it'.[25] As explored in more detail below, these efforts to complicate the relationship between historians and their sources have proven particularly fruitful in the study of mental illness in the past. My own approach to texts about madness and my efforts to form them into a historical narrative have been informed by this scholarship. In this book, a focus on discourse and language seeks to capture the process by which people identified, reacted to, and told stories about madness.

21 Hayden White considers the problem posed by the fact that the historian's own construction of historical narratives is equally embedded in language. See Hayden White 1987.

22 Arnold 2001, p. 7.

23 Rather than following in the footsteps of Emmanuel LeRoy Ladurie, in attempting to remove the Inquisitorial lens to uncover the 'direct testimony of peasants' providing 'an extraordinarily detailed and vivid picture of their everyday life' (Ladurie 1978, p. vii), Arnold 'tr[ies] to examine and understand [...] the conditions that brought about the possibility of this history'. Arnold 2001, p. 3.

24 Beattie 2006, p. 193.

25 Maza 1993, p. 17.

II. Historiography on Madness

In the sixteen years since I first began research into this topic, there has been an increasing interest in considering the social history of madness in the Middle Ages, and several scholars have helped to broaden our view of the subject. After my initial project was completed in 2008, ground-breaking work by Wendy Turner, Elizabeth Mellyn, and Maud Ternon among others further highlighted the ways that legal sources in particular can begin to shed some light on the lived experiences of mad individuals and their communities.[26]

The work of these scholars, appearing in the last decade, has complicated earlier narratives about the treatment of the mad in the Middle Ages. Large-scale histories of mental illness often fell into a narrative either of the triumphalist progress or decline of modern psychiatry. In these narratives, the Middle Ages generally served as a cipher onto which scholars projected either horrific mistreatment or a golden age before the intervention of medicine. The image of the isolated mad individual in the Middle Ages emerged from this debate, particularly in Michel Foucault's *Histoire de la folie à l'age classique*, published in 1961.[27] Foucault's discussion of the discourse of madness remains compelling, even several decades after its initial publication. Ultimately Foucault's main focus is on the development of a system of confinement as part of his larger interest in critiquing the creation of institutional control as a force of modernity. In articulating the relationships between power, knowledge, and control, Foucault is interested in destabilizing the medical model of defining madness in order to demonstrate that it is as much socially constructed as earlier models. He considers the Middle Ages as the starting point from which his history of the medicalization of madness develops, but his desire to create a coherent narrative of change figured as a rupture leads him to idealize the status of the medieval mad as involved in an open 'conversation' with the sane. As he notes in his preface,

> [i]n the Middle Ages, and up until the Renaissance, the debate between man and madness was a dramatic debate that confronted man with the dark powers of the world; and the experience of madness was absorbed in images that spoke of the Fall and the End of All Things, of the Beast, of Metamorphosis, and of all the marvellous secrets of Knowledge. In

26 Turner 2010, Turner 2013a, Mellyn 2014, Ternon 2018.

27 Foucault 1961, Foucault 1972, Foucault 2006.

our time, the experience of madness is made in the calm of a knowledge which, through knowing it too much, passes it over.[28]

Despite his romanticism, the section of Foucault's book that deals with the Middle Ages makes a number of important points about the symbolic value of madness in medieval society, even though his application of that symbolism to real mad people falls short.

Foucault focuses particularly on Sebastian Brant's 1494 *Narrenschiff*, or *Ship of Fools*,[29] arguing that 'among these satirical and novelistic ships, the *Narrenschiff* alone had a genuine existence, for they really did exist, these boats that drifted from one town to another with their senseless cargo'.[30] He elaborates on the literary trope of these ships that 'with a crew of imaginary heroes, moral models or carefully defined social types set out on a great symbolic voyage that brought them, if not fortune, at the very least, the figure of their destiny or of their truth'.[31] Foucault here establishes the symbolic power of the mad as one among many figures that loomed large in the imagination of the late Middle Ages and early Renaissance. In Foucault's analysis, these literary fools represented actual mad people who, especially in Germany, were expelled from towns and set afloat together on ships or sent out on pilgrimages in large groups, becoming 'quite a common sight' on the roads and waterways of their contemporaries.[32]

Foucault acknowledges that some mad people were not expelled, but taken to a 'special place reserved for the detention of the mad', noting that 'only foreign madmen were expelled, and that each town only took responsibility

28 Foucault 2006, pp. xxxiii-xxxiv. The original preface does not appear in the 1972 edition or in any subsequent edition. Foucault 1961, p. iv: 'Au Moyen Âge et jusqu'à la Renaissance, le débat de l'homme avec la démence était un débat dramatique qui l'affrontait aux puissances sourdes du monde ; et l'expérience de la folie s'obnubilait alors dans des images où il était question de la Chute et de l'Accomplissement, de la Bête, de la Métamorphose, et de tous les secrets merveilleux du Savoir. À notre époque, l'expérience de la folie se fait dans le calme d'un savoir qui, de la trop connaître, l'oublie'.

29 Brant 1962.

30 Foucault 2006, p. 9. Foucault 1972, p. 19: 'Mais de tous ces vaisseaux romanesques ou satiriques, le *Narrenschiff* est le seul qui ait eu une existence réelle, car ils ont existé, ces bateaux qui d'une ville à l'autre menaient leur cargaison insensée'.

31 Foucault 2006, p. 8. Foucault 1972, p. 19: 'La mode est à la composition de ces Nefs dont l'équipage de héros imaginaires, de modèles éthiques, ou de types sociaux, s'embarque pour un grand voyage symbolique qui leur apporte sinon la fortune, du moins, la figure de leur destin ou de leur vérité'.

32 Foucault 2006, p. 9. Foucault 1972, p. 19: 'Souvent, les villes d'Europe ont dû voir aborder ces navires de fous'.

for its own citizens who had lost their wits'.[33] Both of these treatments of the mad combine in his depiction of the symbolic value of placing the mad in a liminal social and physical space:

> This enforced navigation is both rigorous division and absolute Passage, serving to underline in real and imaginary terms the *liminal* situation of the mad in medieval society. It was a highly symbolic role, made clear by the mental geography involved, where the madman was *confined at the gates of the cities*. His exclusion was his confinement, and if he had no *prison* other than the *threshold* itself he was still detained at this place of passage.[34]

His image of the mad as simultaneously mentally and physically 'liminal' figures offers a compelling interpretation, suggesting a linkage between the mad person's mental state and his or her social treatment. Indeed, Foucault's ability to elucidate particularly powerful symbols and extrapolate meanings from them provides his most useful legacy. However, since the abridged version of *Histoire de la folie* was first translated into English in 1965, Foucault's work has been both criticized and praised in the Anglophone academy. Many critics argue that he does not provide sufficient evidence to support some of his claims, especially those that cover a wider geographical area.[35] Erik Midelfort, one of the most careful critics of Foucault's historical evidence, found only one recorded instance of an actual ship of fools.[36] More recent

33 Foucault 2006. Foucault 1972, p. 20: 'un lieu de détention réservé aux insensés'; 'On peut donc supposer qu'on ne chasse parmi eux que les étrangers, chaque ville acceptant de se charger seulement de ceux qui sont au nombre de ses citoyens'.

34 Italics in original. Foucault 2006, p. 11. Foucault 1972, p. 22: 'Cette navigation du fou, c'est à la fois le partage rigoureux, et l'absolu Passage. Elle ne fait, en un sens, que développer, tout au long d'une géographie mi-réelle, mi-imaginaire, la situation *liminaire* du fou à l'horizon du souci de l'homme médieval – situation symbolique et réalisée a la fois par le privilège qui est donné au fou d'être *enfermé* aux *portes* de la ville: son exclusion doit l'enclore; s'il ne peut et ne doit avoir d'autre *prison* que le *seuil* lui-même, on retient sur le lieu du passage'.

35 Midelfort 1980, pp. 247–265; Scull 1992, pp. 150–163.

36 Midelfort 1980. Foucault's defenders have cited his much longer and much more heavily-footnoted original French publication to deflect such critiques, arguing that many of the problems other scholars found in his work stem from faulty translation and an inability on their part to read French. On the question of the footnotes, Andrew Scull notes that Foucault was writing from 'intellectual exile' in Sweden, where he lacked access to primary sources and much twentieth century secondary work. Thus, Scull argues, 'Foucault's isolation from the world of facts and scholarship is evident throughout History of Madness. It is as though nearly a century of scholarly work had produced nothing of interest or value for Foucault's project. What interested him, or shielded him, was selectively mined nineteenth-century sources of dubious provenance'. See Scull

research on southern German civic records by Anne Koenig has uncovered significantly more cases, both of temporary confinement of the mad and compulsory movement. When the mad were expelled, in some cases they were sent to family and friends in other towns, but if that was not an option they were sent 'away' more broadly. There is evidence of raftsmen paid to take some 'down the river' but this was done individually, not in a group.[37]

What Foucault ignored in his focus on mad people who were expelled from towns is the significance of the fact that the first resort was always to send them home. Those mad people who traveled on pilgrimages were generally taken there by their families, not sent in large groups of other mad people. Indeed, while some of the literary mad were expelled from society, the literal mad were often cared for in the family home and reincorporated into their previous lives and livelihoods when they were believed to have recovered their sanity. Scholars considering madness in the Middle Ages between the 1970s and the 1990s often followed Foucault's focus on discourse, working to categorize the multiple forms of intellectual discussion about madness. In doing so, they separated the strands of theoretical knowledge, focusing on each one individually.

In 1974, Penelope Doob came out with *Nebuchadnezzar's Children*, and a year later Judith Neaman published *Suggestion of the Devil*.[38] As is clear from their titles, both books considered medieval religious ideas about madness as particularly significant. Doob's study focused strongly on literary texts about madness, while Neaman's concentrated on the various intellectual traditions. Clearly influenced by Foucault's linkage of leprosy and madness, Neaman argued that '[l]epers and madmen, who fell into one social and moral group, were reflections of their diseases, which were

2007. Finally, in 2006, Jonathan Murphy and Jean Khalfa translated the full version, making it more widely available to English-speaking academics. This translation is very conscious of the debate, including all Foucault's original footnotes and carefully translating particularly controversial phrases to provide a defense in translation. To cite one especially pertinent example about the Middle Ages, Foucault asserted 'Les fous alors avaient une existence facilement errante'. (1972, p. 19.) Richard Howard, in the 1965 abridged English edition, translated this as 'Madmen then led an easy wandering existence'. (Foucault 1965, p. 8.) Colin Gordon, in an essay defending Foucault published in 1992, suggested it might be better translated as 'the existence of the mad at that time could easily be a wandering one'. (Gordon 1992, p. 33.) The new translation offers another similar, but even more defensive version by removing the dangerous connotations of 'easy' or 'easily' entirely: 'An itinerant existence was often the lot of the mad'. (Foucault 2006, p. 9.) New translations notwithstanding, the statement is still a problematic one. As Midelfort notes, Foucault's itinerant mad people, traveling from town to town in ships or on the roads, do not appear 'often' in medieval records. (Midelfort 1980, p. 254.)

37 Koenig 2020.

38 Doob 1974, Neaman 1975.

either tests of martyrdom, purgations or punishments for sin'.[39] The two authors cover medieval England, with some forays into French sources, particularly Froissart's chronicle with his account of the madness of Charles VI of France. Carole Rawcliffe, in her overview of medieval English medicine, follows Doob's moral analysis of madness, asserting that 'the insane aroused particular fear and unease because (in theory, at least) their sins seemed so terrible and their punishment so extreme'.[40]

In the early 1990s, two French scholars, Jean-Marie Fritz and Muriel Laharie, argued that in medieval France ideas about madness were polymorphic. Fritz has analyzed medical, theological, and juridical discourses about madness, as well as literary treatments of the mad. He is heavily influenced by Foucault, positing that 'the Foucauldian approach is perfectly suited to the Middle Ages'.[41] The literary focus of Doob and Fritz is unsurprising, given the number of medieval literary figures who exhibit symptoms of mental disturbance, and it is certainly true that the descriptive languages about madness were similar in literary and other texts. However, Stephen Harper may be overstating the case with his contention that '⌊r⌋eal lunatics behaved like literary madmen'.[42] Indeed, Muriel Laharie falls into this assumption as well. She sees the treatment of the mad as part of the growth in the persecution of marginal figures in the twelfth century, describing negative attitudes towards and violence perpetrated against mad people. However, the sources that she uses to demonstrate violent acts against the mad are exclusively literary texts from twelfth-century France.[43] As Sylvia Huot argues, the audience is granted a double perspective on the insane hero in medieval romances: 'When the madman has a character and a personal history, his treatment can be judged as just or unjust'.[44] Thus, the mad figure in romance may be represented as debased and treated violently specifically because of the contrast with his previous exalted state. Much of the work on medieval French literary depictions of madness has focused on the twelfth century. One notable exception is the work of Julie Singer, whose compelling reading of fourteenth- and fifteenth-century literature focuses on the rich metaphorical language used to describe mental function and dysfunction.[45]

39 Neaman 1975, p. 112.
40 Rawcliffe 1995, p. 10.
41 Fritz 1992, p. 4: 'l'approche foucaldienne convient parfaitement à l'âge médiéval'.
42 Harper 2003, p. 62.
43 Laharie 1991, pp. 241–266. She is drawing on the 'persecuting society' posited by Moore 1987.
44 Huot 2003, p. 89.
45 Singer 2018.

Social histories of madness in the Middle Ages have emerged more recently, drawing on a much more extensive and earlier scholarship on the early modern period.[46] In many ways, the focus on the early modern period has been driven by a perceived lack of sources for social histories of madness in the Middle Ages, but recent scholars have found new ways to address that. Social historians have been heavily influenced by the sociological approach of 'labeling theory', which focuses on the importance of language as a tool of social construction. This theory stresses the role of the observer in identifying, comprehending, and describing behavior. The sociologist Erving Goffman, studying asylums in the 1960s, explained how he saw social construction at work:

> Persons who become mental hospital patients vary widely in the kind and degree of illness that a psychiatrist would impute to them, and in the attributes by which laymen would describe them. But once started on the way, they are confronted by some importantly similar circumstances and respond to these in some importantly similar ways. Since those similarities do not come from mental illness, they would seem to occur in spite of it. It is thus a tribute to the power of social forces that the uniform status of mental patient can not only assure an aggregate of persons a common fate and eventually, because of this, a common character, but that this social reworking can be done upon what is perhaps the most obstinate diversity of human materials that can be brought together by society.[47]

Interestingly, Goffman examines the way that these social forces work through narrative. The mental patients he studied created 'an image of [their] life course – past, present, and future – which selects, abstracts,

46 Indeed, early modernists were the first to truly grapple with Foucault's arguments and complicate his narrative. See particularly the essays collected in both volumes of Bynum, Porter, and Shepherd 1985.

47 Goffman 1962, p. 129. For more on labeling theory, see Scheff 1999. Labeling theory has come under considerable criticism for its claims that insanity was solely a social construction, where behaviors were arbitrarily designated as insane by lay people, health professionals, and institutions, a view challenged by other scholars citing biological explanations for mental illness. Although no scholars deny that social construction has a role to play in designations of insanity, the discipline of sociology in particular has chosen to focus on biological explanations. Walter Gove, one particularly vocal proponent of the biological model, argues that 'For all practical purposes, the labeling explanation of mental illness is of historical interest only'. Gove 1979, p. 301. From the historian's perspective, however, the question of the extent to which mental illness is biologically caused versus the extent to which it is socially constructed through the process of labeling is ultimately irrelevant.

and distorts in such a way as to provide [them] with a view of [themselves] that [they] can usefully expound in current situations'.[48] However, these life narratives were consistently deconstructed by the employees of the institution, ranging from nurses to psychiatrists, who challenged the mental patient's interpretation by reasserting the 'truth'.

Historians have found Goffman's work compelling for the ways that it allows them to engage with the social construction found in their narrative sources. The prolific Roy Porter, Michael MacDonald, and Andrew Scull, among others, have studied early modern England, while Erik Midelfort's work has focused on early modern Germany.[49] Michael MacDonald's pioneering analysis of Richard Napier's voluminous case books, in which the physician/astrologer recorded details about his patients and their treatments, is particularly useful for thinking about how madness was understood on a social level. His observations about the crimes committed by mad people are revealing:

> [t]he peculiar nature of much mad crime was that it menaced or destroyed people and property that ought to have been dear to the lunatic. Unreasonable lawbreaking imperiled one's social identity because it attacked the relationships and material objects that situated one in the village community of households and the wider social hierarchy.[50]

Crimes, and indeed legal questions in general, provide much of the available evidence about madness in popular culture, and the nexus between particular criminal actions and madness is significant. This pattern of perceiving the targets of mad crime as inappropriate precisely because they threaten the mad person's membership in the community holds true for medieval France just as it did for early modern England.

In some ways, considerations of the social construction of madness have influenced and in turn have been influenced by new research in disability studies. As I have argued elsewhere, the modern understanding of disability as a politically manifested social identity, like other modern identities, cannot and should not be forcibly laid on the medieval past. Nevertheless, it is fruitful and revealing to use these concepts to think, not about who people were, but about what people did, and, especially in the context of

48 Goffman 1962, p. 150.

49 Andrews and Scull 2003; MacDonald 1981; Midelfort 1994; Midelfort 1999; Porter 1987; Scull, MacKenzie, and Hervey 1996.

50 MacDonald 1981, p. 126.

disability, what they were able to do, what they were allowed to do, and what they were prevented from doing.[51] Mental illness has not always been categorized as a disability in current discourse or in historical accounts. For example, in the medieval section of his *History of Disability*, Henri-Jacques Stiker likens the disabled to the mentally ill, but distinguishes between the two. He sees the disabled, like the fool, as the 'cared-for, integrated marginalized', and traces a Foucauldian trajectory towards confinement, but he does not address the question of madness as a disability.[52]

In her ground-breaking study on medieval disability, Irina Metzler uses religious and medical texts as well as accounts from saints' shrines to examine the treatment of the disabled in medieval culture. Using theories from modern disability studies, she makes a distinction between 'impairment', which she defines as 'a "real", physiological condition' and 'disability', which she calls 'a socially constructed or cultural condition'. In the end, she argues, 'there were very few medieval disabled people'.[53] She suggests that they were economically liminal figures, but she also demonstrates the mechanisms that were put in place, ranging from prostheses like crutches to the cooperation of fellow-travelers, to aid the impaired in reaching their goal of accessing saints' shrines.[54] In her first book, she specifically chose not to discuss mental illness or to address legal aspects of disability, not because she does not see mental illness as part of the larger category, but because she feels that, like leprosy, madness had its own layers of symbolic meaning in the Middle Ages, distinct from other impairments.[55] In her more recent work, Metzler turns her attention to the concept of intellectual disability, arguing that this needs to be studied separately from other kinds of mental incapacity. Her study of normative texts in natural philosophy, theology, and law clearly demonstrates that medieval intellectuals distinguished between mental incapacity that was present from birth and that which was acquired later in life. Nevertheless, they still discussed it in the context of considering mental incapacity in general, and in practice the question of when an individual began to experience it was not always of primary importance.[56] Other

51 Pfau 2010b, p. 96.

52 See Stiker 1999. In current discourse, there is still an uneasy relationship between the physically and the mentally impaired, as addressed by Peter Beresford in an article published in *Disability and Society*, highlighting in particular the need for inclusion. See Beresford 2000.

53 Metzler 2006, p. 6.

54 See Metzler 2006. For other work on disability, see Neugebauer 1996; Stiker 1999; and Turner 2013a.

55 Metzler 2006, p. 6.

56 Metzler 2016.

scholars, including Wendy Turner, working on medieval England where royal wardship cases provide extensive documentation about how madness was defined and how mad people were cared for, have argued that madness more generally can be considered as a disability in this period.[57] This category of disability also leads to questions of social perception and participation. How was madness defined and determined? In what circumstances were people considered mad allowed to interact with others, and in what ways were they socially limited by their perceived illness?

Recent work has demonstrated an increased focus on legal questions about madness. Brendan Parlopiano has provided a thorough study of understandings and treatment of madness in Roman and Canon law. By looking at legal commentary, Parlopiano demonstrates the complexity of medieval ideas about the insanity defense, establishing that '[b]y the fourteenth century then, canonists and civilians alike endorsed the unreserved principle that an insane person, properly proven, could not be held responsible for his or her actions'.[58] Ultimately, Parlopiano, embracing insights from scholars who have focused on evidence of legal practice, brings those studies back to his own analysis of legal theory. He argues that the insane were not expelled from but integrated within society, not only in practice, but also in theory, where 'integration within acceptable limits suffused the concept of insanity; it was part of reflection on the law as well as its practice'.[59] In making this argument, Parlopiano is drawing upon recent work by scholars who have shifted focus from normative texts to legal cases in order to allow access to more nuanced descriptions of madness and its effects on family and community. This work has widened the historical lens beyond the individual to the wider community.

Wendy Turner's wide-ranging work has focused primarily on questions of custody for the mentally incapacitated in England, where from the mid-thirteenth century they became wards of the crown. This created a need for a royal infrastructure that could establish mental incompetence, and evidence of these legal cases survive in the English court rolls. These rich resources provide fascinating evidence of the ways that madness was defined and indeed what was considered necessary mental capacity for functioning in medieval society.[60] Turner also considers a number of legal cases involving crimes committed by people who were, in her terminology, mentally incapacitated.

57 Neugebauer 1996; Turner 2013a.

58 Parlopiano 2013, p. 230.

59 Parlopiano 2013, p. 341.

60 Turner 2013a.

In a larger study of the use of witness testimony in fourteenth- and fifteenth-century French law, Susan Alice McDonough includes a detailed analysis of the case of a woman held captive by her neighbors who argued that they were protecting her because of her insanity.[61] As McDonough notes, the case provides access to a moment of culture clash, where she can see 'two discourses that overlap and yet run in different directions: first, a legal discourse focused on punishing transgressors for laws abridged and with a defined idea of expertise, and second, a vernacular discourse confident in its pragmatic definition of madness with a focus on neighborhood safety, whether or not it met the legal standard'.[62] This case-study approach can be particularly fruitful, as demonstrated by Sara Tilghman Nalle's microhistory of Bartolomé Sánchez, whose Inquisition trial took place between 1553 and 1560 in Cuenca, Spain. As she demonstrates through a careful reading of the record, the Inquisitors struggled to make sense of Sánchez's visions and his claims about his messianic identity. Ultimately, they chose to label him as mentally ill, using the Galenic theory that Nalle notes was experiencing a revival at the time.[63] Both McDonough and Nalle approach their sources with sensitivity, recognizing the ways that legal sources are shaped by the interactions between witnesses, the accused, and representatives of the legal system, and how these interactions can simultaneously reveal and obscure the experiences of individuals and families dealing with the mad.

Elizabeth Mellyn has also been interested in the ways that kin and communities responded to madness and how those responses leave echoes in the legal system. In her study of Florentine judicial records, she works to reveal 'what families, communities, and civic authorities *did* to address the disorder or, in its worst manifestations, the chaos that [madness] visited on their households or unleashed in their streets'.[64] She uncovers the ways that families and communities worked with and through civic authorities to seek resolutions to the problems posed by the mad in both civil and criminal cases. In Florence in the fifteenth and sixteenth centuries that meant that the mad individual was often granted a guardian and sometimes placed in prison. As she notes, these courts became sites 'of social experimentation' where petitioners and officials sought solutions to familial struggles while making space in which 'predators' could 'exploit the vulnerable for their own gain' at the same time.[65]

61 McDonough 2013, pp. 97–121.

62 McDonough 2013, p. 98.

63 Nalle 2001, especially chapter 8.

64 Mellyn 2014, p. 1. Emphasis in the original.

65 Mellyn 2014, p. 5.

Maud Ternon has recently undertaken a similar project for French legal sources. Her work on guardianship cases has shown the ways that French families, like the Florentines studied by Mellyn and the English studied by Turner, used the legal system to control the actions of individuals who were perceived as threatening the patrimony.[66] Through the examination of guardianship cases, Ternon examines the judicial mechanisms whereby decisions limiting an individual's legal capacity to act were put into execution and made public knowledge. In the fourteenth century she finds an increase in recourse to the king's justice in cases of guardianship, driven not by any royal legislation (as we see in England), but rather by demand from the litigants themselves.

All of these scholars have used legal sources to provide an important corrective to the ways that medieval madness had been studied. In each case, criminal records provide a small but significant addition to a larger study of madness and the law. As a result, these works leave space for a deeper consideration of the links between madness and crime, and particularly the ways that individuals could both deploy a language of madness to help comprehend particular criminal acts and seek to ameliorate the damage done to the wider community by those crimes.

III. Structure of the Book

This book seeks to build on the work on legal texts begun by other scholars, by narrowing its focus on the ways that specific narratives about madness and crime reveal the struggles of individuals faced with communal crises. The goal of this book is not to provide a comprehensive consideration of the ways that the mad and their communities interacted with the legal system, on the model of Turner, Mellyn, and Ternon. Rather, it has a more limited and targeted goal of uncovering the understanding and use of madness in a particular source base, the *lettres de remission* ('letters of remission'). As we shall see, these narratives were carefully constructed through a collaborative process between petitioners and royal notaries, and they allow for an in-depth case study of the ways that madness could function as a mechanism for attempting to resolve violent community ruptures.

The texts considered in this book have pointed to a more fluid categorization process in dealing with individual cases than medieval discourses imply. The notaries who were responsible for recording the stories of the

66 Ternon 2018; Ternon 2015.

mad did not force a case to fit into a specific framework, but instead allowed the behavior to be explained with multiple possible reference points. These individuals could be simultaneously described as acting 'like' or 'as though' they were out of their *bonne sens* ('good sense') or *bonne memoire* ('good memory'), frenetic or melancholic, or even possessed. By approaching madness within a particular source base with specific social ramifications, my book calls into question the neat boundaries created by intellectual historians. In practice, the definition of and the need to cope with the mad caused medieval people to embrace a large number of potentially conflicting frameworks in order to understand them and arrive at pragmatic solutions. People whose behavior did not fit into expected patterns, often through violent or excessive manifestations, could be considered mad, but that was not the only possible interpretation of their behavior. On the level of theologians and physicians, such concepts as melancholy, frenzy, possession, witchcraft, and folly were mutually exclusive. However, when faced with unusual, inexplicable behavior, medieval people often used many combinations of these terms to try to explain the problem. Madness as a category, much like today, could cover anything from making a foolish decision to a frenetic fury leading to murder.

Historical records showing how people identified madness and sought to understand and respond to it particularly lend themselves to considering social construction. The texts used for this book describe social interactions and the ways they were interpreted by participants and observers. These interactions are necessarily mediated, and may tell us very little about the 'reality' of the events and the conditions depicted. Nevertheless, the texts provide a great deal of information about how certain behaviors could lead communities to identify individuals as mad, who was involved in providing that identification, what kinds of and how many 'proofs' were expected in order to confirm that identification, and what mechanisms were available for treating or coping with a person who had been identified as mad. Ultimately, the language of madness provided a space through which ruptured communities could be, at least on the surface, repaired.

Between 1364 and 1498, the king's chancery filled one hundred and thirty-four registers, containing 52,622 acts, of which 38,860 are letters of remission, or seventy-four percent of the total.[67] From this large base, I selected a sampling of thirty-five registers to search, around a quarter of

67 These numbers are my own calculations. They differ slightly from those in the study by Michel François. He found 52,698 total acts and 38,655 remission letters. The difference is minimal, and may be due to some typographical errors in his article, most notably when he

the total, containing 13,671 acts, 9,852 of which are remission letters. In addition, I gleaned a few other letters from the regional indices and editions available.[68] My sampling garnered one hundred fifty-five letters that mention madness, comprising one percent of the total letters read. These letters are scattered throughout the registers, not clustered around particular dates, suggesting that mental illness was not a common trope in the genre but a relatively unusual manifestation for the royal notaries who recorded and helped to compose these letters.

There were many ways to write a letter of remission in the fourteenth and fifteenth centuries. There was no need to prove a lack of guilt in remission letters, although many did strive to do so, and it was certainly not necessary to invent circumstances that would exculpate the accused. Even if an attempt was made to provide extenuating circumstances for the crime, generally the letters were focused on the bad reputation of the victim or the crime was explained as an accident. The invocation of madness was not necessary and, in some cases, could lead to further difficulties, since some letters included a caveat requiring the person to be kept under guard as a condition for pardon.[69] Indeed, claims of mental disturbance appear in the archives rarely, but consistently, over the one hundred fifty year period under examination here. On average, letters about madness appear in one percent of the total remission letters in a book, and in the books that were fully examined they never exceeded three percent. On the other hand, only two of the thirty-five books searched yielded no references to mental illness. Thus, the choice to mention madness appears to have been a conscious one, and there is little likelihood that the notaries developed a standard form for writing about it, the way they appear to have for writing about tavern brawls. Instead, the choice to explain a crime in terms of mental disturbance was a difficult and potentially damaging one.

Chapter One delves into the complexities of language about madness through an examination of the intellectual context within which the royal notaries were working. Legal discourse about madness engaged with questions of responsibility, governance, culpability, and punishment. Legal texts conceived of mental illness as an inability to comprehend, and therefore a propensity to infringe upon, the rules governing social and legal interactions.

lists AN JJ 204 as containing 116 total acts, of which 120 are remission letters. In that register I found there were in fact 136 total acts. See François 1942, 317–324.

68 Chevalier 1993; Dossat, LeMason, and Wolff 1983; Guérin 1909; Gut 2000; Le Cacheux 1907–1908; Petit-Dutaillis 1908; Samaran 1966.

69 For example, at the end of AN JJ 173 fo 33v no 63 (in 1425).

The threat to order that mad people represented was therefore twofold: they could not be trusted to care for themselves or their own property, and they might not respect other people's lives or properties. Because the mad did not understand what they did, they were not held responsible for any contracts into which they entered. However, law codes reveal an uncertainty about mad criminals. Although all the legal texts agreed that the mad should not be punished for crimes, the explanations for their immunity differed, often within a single text. This ambiguity may have contributed to a need for royal intervention into such cases, which manifested in the form of the king's remission for crime. The royal notaries were not solely influenced by legal terminology and concepts, however. The language they used to describe madness pulled from a wide variety of discourses in order to present a fuller understanding of the meaning of mental incapacity.

Chapter Two examines the narratives in remission letters to consider how the family advocated for the mad person by constructing stories about the crime, but also about the person's entire life. The evidence provided for mental illness earlier in the person's life was often idiosyncratic, and sometimes the narratives tried to provide logical linkages between the earlier behavior and the ultimate crime of the mad person. These individual narratives reveal a wide spectrum of beliefs about what caused madness and what kinds of behaviors and criminal acts were coded as mad. Although each narrative was distinct, a clear pattern emerges whereby the actions of the individual identified as mad disrupt familial and communal bonds.

Chapter Three discusses the evidence in these letters for community and family actions, examining the networks available to help or hinder the mad. As noted in Chapter Two, the crimes of the mentally ill most often targeted their kin and communal ties, rupturing the identity of the criminal. Through the medium of remission letters, these ties were reformed, and connections were reconstructed. The family and the community simultaneously wished to aid the mad and feared the possible consequences of insanity. The mentally ill were sometimes taken to saints' shrines to seek cures, but often they were kept in chains or otherwise guarded. The remission letters also often sought to tell the story from the perspective of the criminal, thereby encouraging the family members and the notary composing the letter to attempt to rationalize the insanity, creating an alternative understanding of reality through which the mad person's crime was comprehensible.

As Jehan le Vignon's case suggests, madness was generally determined through acts that were identified by other people, and generally disrupted expectations of kin and communal rights and responsibilities. The disease was not marked on the body, and the mad did not make up minority communities within the larger whole. Insanity could appear at any point during an individual's lifespan, and could happen to any person. Indeed, in the late fourteenth and early fifteenth centuries it affected the French king himself. Madness could be cyclical, as people who were mad for a time could suddenly become sane and vice versa. Yet, rather than being expelled, the mentally ill were generally reincorporated into these networks they had ruptured. During periods of sanity, most people were allowed to resume their normal lives and engage in their usual activities and duties. The very instability of the mad identity and the investment of the community make these narratives about madness particularly rich and compelling. Despite the ways in which madness was imagined in terms of interiority and individuality, in the end all these discussions returned to the implications of madness: how the singular mad person affected and was affected by the larger community.

Through a close examination of these sources we can begin to unpack the complexity of the individual stories told. Though we can never truly access lived experiences, in these carefully constructed narratives about the actions of people labeled as mad, we can get a glimpse of the efforts and struggles of families and communities both to understand and to cope with the repercussions of these actions. The positive note of familial and communal solidarity in rallying around the mad individual is often belied within the main narrative that reveals the difficulties of dealing with mad family members. In this way, the narrative structure of remission letters about the mad are similar to fairytale structures as elucidated by Marina Warner. Critics of fairytales often suggest that they create an unrealistic view of marriage as a perfect state, but Warner argues that the structure of the 'happily ever after' conclusion in a wedding 'masks the fact that many stories picture the conditions of marriage during the course of their telling' and not in positive terms. Instead the 'glib promise of [fairytales'] traditional ending' is set against the background of 'the knowledge of misery within marriage that the preceding story reveals in its every line'.[70] Similarly, remission letters imagine the reconstruction of a community by reintegrating the very person who had ruptured it in the first place. However, within the narrative we can see the cracks of that community, the pressures put on individuals to fulfill the expectations of others, the ways that families struggled to provide household care, and the consequences of failure on multiple levels. The promise of the narrative, that the friends and family of the mad individual will care for him or her in future, is undermined by the

70 Warner 1994, pp. 217–219.

story that has already been told, just as the fairytale promise of 'happily ever after' rests on a blithe dismissal of the rest of the tale. In telling their story publicly to their neighbors, remission seekers invoked that same power of words to reframe and reconfigure their hopes for the future, denying their knowledge of the more likely outcome based on the past. Despite the clear evidence of the struggles and challenges of coping with mad people in the community, these remission seekers still planned to continue their efforts.

1. Composing Communities

Languages of Madness in Remission Letters

Abstract
An examination of the intellectual context within which the royal notaries worked sheds light on the complex layers of language about madness in the fourteenth and fifteenth centuries. Legal texts conceived of mental illness as an inability to comprehend, and therefore a propensity to infringe upon, the rules governing social and legal interactions. The royal notaries were not solely influenced by legal terminology and concepts, however. The language they used to describe madness pulled from a wide variety of discourses to present a fuller understanding of the meaning of mental incapacity. Unlike scholars writing within a single discourse, however, notaries often combined terms in an effort to express their particular image of madness.

Keyterms: Remission, Notaries, Translation, Language

When Jehannecte Troppé murdered her husband, Thomas Baillet, her 'relatives and immediate family'[1] sought a letter of remission for her. Jehannecte herself was unable to join them since she was in prison in the town of Bayeux at the time. Two months after the murder the family traveled about 153 miles (247 kilometers) from Bayeux to Paris,[2] where the duke of Bedford was holding the position of Regent for the two-year-old English king of France, Henry. There, Jehannecte's family, which probably included her father Thomas, mentioned by name in the letter, met with the royal notary, Jean de Rinel. With his help, the family composed a letter explaining Jehannecte's crime and asking that she be pardoned.[3] It is impossible to know whether the Troppé family arrived

1 AN JJ 173 no 63 fo 33v. Edited in Le Cacheux 1907–1908, pp. 181–183: 'parens et amis'. See Gauvard 1991, pp. 643–651 for a discussion of the meaning of 'parens et amis charnels'.

2 The trip would have taken around three days on a horse or nine or more days on foot. For an estimate of travel time I used Dunn and Davidson 2000, p. 487

3 For more on these documents, see Davis 1987, pp. 7–25; Gauvard 1991, vol. 1, pp. 59–110.

Pfau, A., *Medieval Communities and the Mad: Narratives of Crime and Mental Illness in Late Medieval France*. Taylor & Francis Group, 2021
DOI: 10.5117/9789462983359_CH01

in Paris intending to mention that Jehannecte was mad or whether they came to that decision through consultation with the notary Jean de Rinel, but it is clear that the letter was composed with madness as the central theme.

According to the letter, one night about fifteen days before the feast of All Saints in 1424, Jehannecte got up out of bed and began destroying her clothes, their pots and pans, and all the other household items that she could find. The next day, she opened a bag of bread flour and scattered it around the house, refusing to tell her husband why. Thomas Baillet hoped his wife would stop this behavior and they could live 'peaceably together, as they had been always since their marriage'.[4] On the night of 4 November, Jehannecte, her husband, and her eleven-year-old brother were lying in bed together when she picked up a rock and hit her husband on the head several times, then got back into bed beside him. When Thomas Baillet was able to speak, he told her to light the candle. Jehannecte had to go to a neighbor's house in order to find fire, even though they had covered their own when they went to bed. When she saw her husband's wounds, Jehannecte was shocked and had no idea that she had caused them. However, when Thomas Baillet died eight days later, she was arrested and put in prison in Bayeux, where, as her family claimed, she and the child with which she was pregnant were in danger of dying. These were the basic points of the story that the family told, but the way that they told it framed the narrative in terms of madness. Having made the choice to describe Jehannecte's crime in this way, the supplicants and the notary had to find or create an acceptable shared language and understanding of madness with which to do so.[5] Whereas Jean de Rinel was literate, Latinate, and licensed in the law, the letter was composed in French and would be read aloud to the community where Jehannecte Troppé was in prison.

I. Letters of Remission

The first letters of remission appeared in the records of the French king's chancery at the beginning of the fourteenth century.[6] The earliest of these letters were mostly granted to people who claimed to have been falsely

4 AN JJ 173 no 63 fo 33v. Edited in Le Cacheux 1907–1908, pp. 181–183: 'se tenissent paisiblement ensemble, come ilz avoient esté tousjours depuis leur mariage'.

5 In this study of the vernacular French vocabularies of madness, I am inspired in part by Helmut Puff's proviso that what is significant 'is not language in its abstraction', but instead 'the ways in which historical actors, magistrates, officials, translators, redactors, experts, or defendants used language'. Puff 2003, p. 3.

6 The first remission letter appeared in May of 1304. See Gauvard 1991, vol. 1, 64.

accused or to forgive members of the nobility who had been engaged in warfare that was not sanctioned by the king.[7] Over time, letters were also granted to non-nobles as a pardon for crimes they had committed. Through this development, the French king made a number of interrelated claims about his power and authority.[8] With these letters, the king was exercising his powers of grace and mercy by choosing to grant life instead of death to his erring subjects. His mercy did not reflect justice, but, like God's mercy established in the promise of the New Testament, it acted above human perceptions of punishment as a direct correlation to crime.[9] Indeed, this understanding of remission is written into the framing text that surrounded the individual stories about crimes. The letter was written in the king's voice, and the act of remission was a recorded speech act, where the king said, 'We, preferring mercy to the rigor of justice [...], grant remission'.[10] On a lower plane, remission letters demonstrated the king's power to override the execution of justice in his realm, thus making him the equal of the Emperor.[11] As these related concepts of mercy and authority demonstrate, remission was not about justice but about power. The king could and did act above the law in granting pardons, and there was no need for petitioners to establish their innocence. Most of the petitioners admitted their guilt, much as they might in a confession to a man of God, but they were careful to establish that the crime was unusual, and not part of a criminal lifestyle. The king was gracious in his mercy, granting remission for treason, and even in some cases pardoning an individual for a crime for which his or her partner had already been executed.[12]

7 Some of these early letters can be found edited at numbers 3759, 3914, 3986, 4054, 4177, 4231, 4322, 4357, 4603, 4767, 4788, 4841, and 5101 in Jassemin and Vallée 1999, vol. 2. See also Justine Firnhaber-Baker's work on the subject of private warfare through the examination of remission letters. Firnhaber-Baker 2014; Firnhaber-Baker 2007; Firnhaber-Baker 2006.

8 It has been argued that the fourteenth century saw an increased effort on the part of the king to demonstrate his power through the legal system. Brissaud 1971, pp. 552–556; Cohen 1993, p. 51.

9 Thus, Alexander Murray is mistaken when he argues that 'A Letter of Remission, by definition, declared its beneficiary not guilty'. Rather, a letter of remission, like the remission granted by a priest to whom a person confessed, pardoned the beneficiary whether or not the beneficiary had committed the crime of which he or she was accused. Murray 1998, vol. 1, p. 207.

10 'voulans misericorde preferer a rigueur de justice anous[...]quicte remis et pardonne'. This exact phrasing may not appear in all letters, but it is a common choice to represent this sentiment, which is certainly present in all of them.

11 Texier 1999, p. 348. For more on the development of the legal concept of the king as emperor in his realm in the thirteenth century, see Voegelin 1997, vol. 3, p. 60.

12 During the reign of Charles V, the definition of *lèse-majesté* was broadened to incorporate verbal as well as physical injuries to the king and to the rest of the royal line. See Hoareau-Dodinau

The development of remission letters as an outlet for royal authority made them an increasingly central occupation of the king's chancery over time. While they began as a very small percentage of the chancery output (between 0 and 2 percent from 1304 to 1338), in the 1340s there was a sudden increase in production such that they made up fully a quarter of the chancery records. In the 1350s the percentage rose to about half, then again to around three-quarters in the 1370s. The percentage held relatively steady at 75, with a few spikes every ten years or so, when some books record 90 percent or more remission letters. The percentage of output did not fall until the 1480s, when it began averaging half of chancery production again.[13] Remission was limited to capital crimes, but during the height of the popularity of the letters they were granted for a wide range of criminal acts including counterfeiting currency, suicide, bestiality, theft, and rape, all of which could carry a death penalty but did not necessarily do so. There were attempts to limit the range of crimes for which remission could be granted, but apart from the exclusion of suicide from the mid-fifteenth century, these reforming efforts were largely unsuccessful until the sixteenth century, which is outside the range of this study.[14]

Several scholars have shown that, from the perspective of the king, remission letters demonstrated his jurisdictional power. Through granting mercy, the king exercised his ability to override the local legal traditions and the jurisdictional powers of both secular and religious lords.[15] As a result, the letter itself was embedded within a language of royal power. Each letter

2002, p. 204. For examples of individuals who were granted remission after their compatriots were executed, see Cohen 1990, pp. 285–286.

13 The rest of the chancery documents are made up of ordonnances, letters of anoblissement, letters of naturalité, amortissements, concession or confirmation of privileges, and letters of abolition. For a table with the numbers of remission letters and the numbers of total acts, see François 1942. Although I found some of his counting to be questionable (particularly for AN JJ 189 and AN JJ 204, where the number of remission letters exceeds the number of total acts), my own counting resulted in numbers close enough to his to allow these percentages to stand. Note that Claude Gauvard uses these same numbers to argue that the granting of remission letters decreased due to criticism in 1400. See the table in Gauvard 1991, vol. 1, p. 65. Although numerically it is true that there were fewer remission letters granted, I think this can be traced rather to lower chancery work during a time when France was suffering from civil war and English invasion. Remission letters remain a high percentage of chancery output during this time. In fact, the only true gap in the granting of remission appears between 1434 and 1441 (the gap occurs between AN JJ 175 and AN JJ 176), when Charles VII was in the process of taking Paris from the English.

14 Davis notes that in the sixteenth century the vast majority of letters of remission were for murder. Davis 1987, p. 7.

15 Gauvard 1991; Texier 2001; Texier 1999.

began with the name of the king, 'by the grace of God, king of France',[16] and ended with formulaic language that reiterated the letter's function as a speech act that granted remission through the king's sovereign power. The letters operated as both written and oral acts of power, since they had to be carried back and read aloud in the local courts to be fully legitimized, thus transferring this notion of royal power from the center to the periphery. The letter was framed within an expression of the king's power, so that it simultaneously fulfilled the functions of pardoning a particular individual and, through the particular rhetoric of the letter, using that pardon to reinforce the king's sovereignty. For example, in a letter from 1387 composed on behalf of Robert Layné, a poor man whose madness caused him to say that he would fight anyone, including the king, Charles VI granted him remission by saying,

> wishing to extend to him Our grace and mercy, We have assuredly considered these things. Desiring mercy to be [...] preferred to the rigor of justice, to this supplicant in the case above said we have acquitted, remitted, and pardoned all punishment and offense, criminal, corporal and civil that he has or could have justly incurred for the act and occasion of the said words, by him thus said, and through this present [letter] by special grace, full power and royal authority we do acquit, remit and pardon and restore him to his good reputation and renown in the country, and to his goods non-confiscated, and we impose on this [topic] perpetual silence in the present and in the future by Our procurer and by all our other officers.[17]

This coda, which is repeated in variations in every letter, expressed the power of the king to erase the criminal act committed by the pardoned individual. The irony of this reinforcement of kingly power embedded within a generous gesture of pardon for treasonous speech only increases its force. The king demonstrated his grace and mercy, which extended directly from his particular role as king of France by the grace of God.

16 'Par la grace de dieu, Roy de France'.

17 Saunier 1993, p. 498: 'nous lui vueillons eslargir Notre grâce et miséricorde Nous a de certes ses choses considérées voulans miséricorde estre miséricorde estre (sic) préférée à rigeur de justice à ycellui suppliant ou cas dessus dit toute peine offense criminele corporelle et civile qu'il a ou peut avoir encouru envers justice pour le fait et occasion des dictes paroles par lui ainsi dictes avons quitté, remis et pardonné et par ces présentes de grâce espécial pleine puissance et auctorité royal quittons, remettons et pardonnons et le restituons à sa bonne fame renommée au pays et à ses biens non confisquez et imposons sur ce silence perpétuel par Notre procureur présent et à venir et à touz autres noz officiers'.

Perhaps the strongest evidence that remission letters were seen as a way of advertising power is the continuity of the granting of pardons. During the English 'occupation' of France, the chancery continued to grant remission on behalf of Henry, 'by the grace of God, king of France and England'.[18] Jehannecte Troppé's letter was composed during this period. The dukes of Burgundy, further proving that the ability to grant pardon was seen as a significant part of the power of government, wielded this power in their own territories.[19] Enclosed within this rhetorical expression of the king's sovereign power and majesty was the story of the particular crime the king had pardoned.

The path to any remission letter began with a crime. In Jehannecte Troppé's case, this would be the murder of Thomas Baillet. From this starting point, there were many possible peregrinations that would lead to the ultimate decision to seek the king's pardon. Sometimes, as happened to Jehannecte, the accused would have been imprisoned, and would either choose to acquire a letter before the trial took place or after having been found guilty. In other cases, the accused might have left town, essentially going into self-imposed exile, since medieval French courts considered flight as proof of guilt.[20] A third possible route was preventive pardon, where the accused had neither been arrested nor fled the scene, but wanted to have the reassurance of pardon on the chance that the case might be pursued. Although some letters insisted on the innocence of the supplicant, most supplicants admitted to their guilt. The process of receiving the king's pardon was both time-consuming and expensive. First a petitioner had to travel to the king's council, which could be difficult, particularly for people who did not live in or around Paris, a fact reflected in the general geographic scope of the letters copied by the king's chancery. Indeed, the king's own travel impacted the letters received and ratified, since some letters relating to crimes committed many years before were recorded when the king happened to pass through the area.[21] The king, or more likely an officer of the

18 See the letters collected in Longnon 1878: 'par la grace de Dieu roy de France et d'Angleterre'. See also those collected in Le Cacheux 1907–1908, vol. 1.

19 For more on Burgundian pardons, see Arnade and Prevenier 2015, which also includes some edited and translated letters, though none pertaining to madness. More of the letters have been collected and edited (though not translated) in Petit-Dutaillis 1908.

20 Indeed, in this sense, remission letters act as a kind of 'passport', allowing the recipient to return. Much like medieval passports, the power was in the king's seal. For more on the development of the paperwork of identity, see Groebner 2007.

21 One of these, in AN JJ 99 fo 25 (in 1367), is a remission for a crime committed forty years earlier. The existence of these letters raises interesting questions about administration of the law in this period. If in some cases a person could commit a crime and then wait thirty years

chancery, would then command a royal notary, together with the accused or the family members of the accused, to compose a letter explaining the circumstances leading up to the crime and telling the story of the crime itself. To be ratified, the letter had to be read before the king's council. Assuming it was satisfactory, the council would provide the remission seeker with a seal. For an extra fee, the letter would also be recorded in the official record by the chancery scribes, so that there was an external source proving the existence of the pardon.[22] The price of the whole process was officially set at thirty-two Parisian sous in the fourteenth century: six for the redaction, six for the seal, and twenty for the registration in the chancery's books.[23] This was more than a week's wages for most artisans,[24] and although the king tried to control the price by passing ordinances, the ultimate tally could be much higher, particularly when the cost of a journey to Paris and accommodation while seeking pardon are added to the consideration. This was not the end of the process, however, since the petitioner had to return to the jurisdiction in which the crime had been committed and give the letter to the local administrator of justice. The letter would then be read aloud in the presence of the adverse party, who could be the bereaved family of a murder victim or the neighbors who brought the case to the attention of the court. If someone raised an objection the remission could be annulled, taking the accused back to the beginning.[25]

In theory, remission from crime was available to any criminal who had committed a capital crime, was able to bring his or her case before the king's council, and whose case appealed to the king's desire to practice lenient justice. In practice, remission letters had a number of overlapping goals which affected the rhetoric of the letter. The letter reflected the agendas of both the king and the individual seeking remission, each of which was refracted through the interpretive framework of the royal notaries who

before deciding to seek remission when the king was handily in the area, then what conditions were necessary for someone to be legally pursued?

22 Christian Gut 2000 provides a diplomatic study of the documents themselves.

23 Gauvard 1991, vol. 1, p. 68.

24 Geremek 1968, pp. 90–94. Geremek provides the day wages of masons, carpenters, and their assistants as an example, noting in one case from the early fourteenth century that masons and carpenters were paid 4 sous a day, while their assistants were paid 2 sous. He also notes that the day wages were seasonal, since the combined earnings of one carpenter and his valet in the late fourteenth century were 5 sous a day during summer, but only 4 sous a day during winter, presumably reflecting the change in available working hours as the days got shorter.

25 Some letters demonstrate this practice, since they appear in multiple versions in the chancery archives.

wrote the letter down.[26] Thus, there was no single author for a remission letter: it was a cooperative process. This was particularly true for remission letters for mad people, which were generally sought not by the accused but by their relatives and close family members. Jehannecte Troppé's letter, as noted above, was sought by her father and other relatives. The letters for the mad therefore reflect the multiple perspectives of the mad person's relatives and the scribe. It is more appropriate to think of these letters as 'composed' rather than 'authored'.

Historians have long recognized the value of remission letters, but until recently, most have mined the letters for anecdotal evidence, deconstructing the narratives in order to use them to construct other narratives. Natalie Zemon Davis's book about remission letters, *Fiction in the Archives*, focused scholarly attention on the ways these narratives about crime were constructed.[27] Unlike the title of the work, which unfortunately has been misinterpreted by some scholars to mean these sources cannot be used by historians,[28] the book itself does not seek to destroy the value of the texts but to focus historians' attention on their narratives, rather than on searching them for data. Like all historical sources, remission letters are not reflections of a factual reality that can be uncovered, but were constructed with a particular goal and include such information as is pertinent to that goal, formed into a coherent narrative thread. Although Davis never insists on the letters' fictionality as opposed to a possible 'true' event, she shows the ways in which these letters were written using familiar narrative devices that, to her, sprang from a shared knowledge of storytelling techniques.[29] Brian Stock observes that 'stories do not convince us by their arguments but by their lifelikeness [...]. They may be verifiable, if we can get at the "facts"; but mainly they are believable'.[30] The composers of remission letters would have been familiar with the process of creating a personal narrative of an event from storytelling and confession, which remission letters closely resemble. Where confession creates a moralized story within the context of an omniscient God, remission moralizes within the context of a king

26 Our knowledge of the royal notaries becomes significantly more complete in the seventeenth century, but for some details about them in the fifteenth century, see Lapeyre and Scheurer 1978, vol. 1, especially the introduction by Robert-Henri Bautier, ix-xxxix.

27 Davis 1987.

28 This became clear to me in the question and answer sessions of a number of conference panels in which I participated, when members of the audience were 'surprised' to learn that remission letters were not merely 'fiction in the archives'.

29 Davis 1987.

30 Stock 1990, p. 11.

who provides justice, but could, like God, be convinced to temper it with mercy.[31] It is essential to recognize and explore the ways in which these letters were constructed, who was involved in their redaction, and what kinds of discourses these composers pulled from to create their narratives.

More recent work on remission letters, particularly in France, has been influenced by Davis's focus on narratives, and has tried to understand these texts on their own terms.[32] Claude Gauvard's study of letters from the fourteenth and fifteenth centuries focuses on the way that these narratives reflect social perceptions of crime and criminal behavior. Through statistical analysis of the letters, she demonstrates the relationship between particular social roles and types of crimes.[33] Her evidence shows that madness was only used in one percent of remission letters.[34] Gauvard notes that the actions of the mad as reported in remission letters 'contrasts sharply with normality',[35] causing the close family and relatives involved in the remission letter to express astonishment; in her extensive study of crime she does not have space to analyze this astonishment or the behavior that elicited it, however. In looking at the treatment of madness in medieval English courts, Barbara Hanawalt similarly argues that '[a]ll the cases of mental disorder described in the rolls seem to have been the sort that would be readily recognizable to the average person: abnormalities as obvious as attempted suicide, bizarre behavior, and motiveless violence'.[36] While I cannot speak for the English legal documents Hanawalt refers to, in the French remission letters I have examined, the violence is not always 'motiveless'. Indeed, a woman who attacks or even kills her husband because she believes that he was unfaithful, however wrong she may have been, does not seem motiveless to a modern reader.[37] If the family of such a woman in the Middle Ages believed this

31 Hayden White sees historical narrative as intimately attached to moralizing. See Hayden White 1980. While others have challenged his assertion that moralism is the only grounds on which a narrative can be given a conclusion, notably Mink 1981, it is certainly true that the personal narratives in remission letters are intimately connected to a legal sensibility and a moralizing perspective.

32 See especially Gauvard 1991; Gauvard, 1995; Hoareau-Dodinau 1999; Saunier 1993; Texier 1999.

33 Gauvard 1991.

34 Gauvard 1991, vol. 1, p. 436. My own research has confirmed this number. While Davis notes that madness was one of the eleven cases in which murder was pardonable by the king, she does not discuss how madness was elaborated in the letters of remission. Davis 1987, p. 12n.

35 Gauvard, 1991, vol. 1, 437: 'tranchent sur la normalité'.

36 Hanawalt 1979, p. 148.

37 There are several letters that revolve around spousal jealousy and madness, as I discuss in more detail below. See especially AN JJ 173 fo 33v no 63 (in 1425) (edited in Le Cacheux 1907–1908,

kind of violent behavior had to be explained by the onset of madness, then it is interesting for the very fact that it would not be recognizable to the 'average person' today, but would have been to the 'average person' of the fourteenth century.

Annie Saunier's essay on madness in the remission letters does an excellent job of examining two particular letters, but her small sample size limited the kinds of observations she was able to make.[38] The two letters she focuses on are both unusual cases. The first letter described a man who had gone mad from old age, recovered his sanity, and then had a relapse during which he murdered his wife. The letter is unusual in its brevity, disposing of the details of the case in seven lines of the manuscript, filling the rest of the letter with the rhetoric of the king's pardon.[39] In the second letter, the mad man was rescued by local nobles who called in a physician to help him,[40] providing the only case out of the 155 letters I have examined where a physician's aid was sought for a mad person. Maud Ternon, whose chapters on remission letters draw extensively from my own research, is also focused on exploring the ways these narratives can show us what people thought about mental illness. Ternon's work provides an excellent overview, but she generally draws details from multiple letters rather than looking at the flow of an individual narrative in depth.[41]

Remission letters were detailed stories, carefully constructed to gain pardon without changing the perceived truth too much. Pascal Texier argues that remission letters, despite the royal notary's influence, express the 'subjectivity' and 'manner of speaking' of the supplicant.[42] It is important to recognize, however, that, as with all legal records, these are not unmediated voices. Although the words of the supplicant are, indeed, present, they have been redacted to an appropriate form through a cooperative effort with the notary, who knew what kinds of questions to ask and what kind of information was necessary to the letter. Texier's hopeful reading of the

pp. 181-183); AN JJ 146 fo 83v no 162 (in 1394); AN JJ 173 fo 188v no 392 (in 1426) (edited mistakenly as JJ 175 no 392 in Longnon 1878, p. 208); and AN JJ 173 fo 168 no 349 (in 1425).

38 Saunier 1993.

39 AN JJ 130 fo 118v no 217 (in 1387), edited in Saunier 1993, 497–498.

40 AN JJ 131 fo 103 no 166 (in 1387), edited in Saunier 1993, 498–499.

41 Ternon 2018.

42 Texier elaborates 'à travers la mise en forme écrite par un clerc, c'est en tout premier lieu le point de vue du rémissionnaire qui est exprimé: ce sont donc sa subjectivité et sa manière de dire qui nous sont restitués pour l'essentiel. L'objet de la présente communication est donc d'analyser comment le rémissionnaire joue avec les concepts de responsabilité ou de culpabilité, et quelles stratégies il est amené à développer pour obtenir sa grâce'. 2001, p. 482.

letters does not allow for the complexity of the interactions involved in the creation of these documents.

The narratives of remission letters each follow their own pattern to describe the individual's life. The terms used to describe madness and some of the themes of the narratives often follow familiar lines, but the letters are not formulae into which details are placed. Rather, each narrative was specific to the person about whom the letter was written, and created constructs of normal and transgressive behavior around which to describe the case. Composers of remission letters sought to create narrative coherence within the story of a particular person's life. While letters for sane criminals generally focused on the single day of the crime, letters for the mad often returned to earlier evidence of madness, describing the first remembered incidence of mad behavior and any others recalled in the intervening years.

The pattern of the genre of remission letters began to develop in the mid-fourteenth century. Certain information was considered necessary to the genre, while other structural elements were added over time. For example, only fifty-four of the one hundred fifty-five letters examined for this study included the age of the supplicant. By the mid-fifteenth century, although many of the letters still lacked the age, in some letters the royal notaries left a blank space where the age would normally appear in the composition.[43] In her examination of nineteenth-century settlement examinations under the English Poor Laws, Carolyn Steedman argues that from their inception in the seventeenth century, these 'enforced narratives' developed a formulaic pattern based on what was considered necessary information in describing the life of a poor servant for the purposes of determining whether or not he or she was eligible for poor relief in a certain village.[44] The narratives produced conceal the process of question and answer that provided the necessary information, much as remission letters conceal the collaboration between notary and supplicant that together created the final product, in which certain information is considered necessary and other details are left out.

43 The earliest ones I found came from Charles VII's reign, in AN JJ 182-188. During the same period, other details also became part of the expected formula. AN JJ 187 fo 138v no 252 (in 1455) leaves a blank for the town in which the supplicant lived, AN JJ 182 fo 51v no 86 (in 1453) leaves a blank for the day on which the events occurred, and AN JJ 199 fo 134v no 129 (in 1463), interestingly, leaves a blank space for the name of the man who was murdered.

44 Steedman 2002. Thank you to Kali Israel for pointing out how Steedman's work could be useful for my own. For a similar kind of construction of proof in the medieval period, see Rosenthal 2003.

Because the letters enacted the king's mercy, some of the personal information about the supplicants was clearly intended to demonstrate their status as worthy recipients of that mercy. Many of them fit a particular mold of deserving supplicants described as 'poor' people, often 'laborers with their arms', who were responsible for their spouses, children, and sometimes aged parents. It was, of course, not always possible to fit each supplicant into this particular pattern, but all of them were described as being of *bonne fame et renomée*, or 'good reputation and renown', before the singular occurrence of the criminal act for which they sought remission. If the supplicant was not of good reputation before the particular crime, any other crime or infraction he or she was accused of had to be listed within the letter that then would note that the supplicant was of good reputation with the exception of those cases.[45]

The moment of crime acts as the climax of a narrative that humbly requests (although, because only successful letters were recorded in the chancery archives, in all the letters examined here this request has already been granted) the action of the king in a future moment outside the bounds of the narration. While the granting of remission is the intended end of the story within the text, it is not the only possible ending presented by the narrator, who envisions the likelihood of death in prison while awaiting trial, a trial that leads to execution, or a permanent, self-imposed exile. The moral thrust of the narrative is that the king's law is just but also merciful, and that, unlike his anonymously bureaucratic courts, he himself is willing to consider cases on an individual, personal level. In fact, this distinction is purely rhetorical, which must have been eminently clear to the king's subjects during periods of regency, particularly the regency for Henry, the English king, who was a baby at his coronation. Instead of indicating a personal acquaintance with the woes of his subject, the French king's granting of remission was in fact the bureaucratic royal system functioning in full force.[46]

Many of the letters composed for mad people began from the rhetorical premise that they were not written from the perspective of the mad criminal. Instead, in most cases, letters for mad people came from their *parens et amis*

45 This most often occurred within letters written for soldiers, who sought remission for a long list of campaign-related crimes, such as looting, pillaging, and raping. This is true in several of the earliest letters of remission, which can be found edited in Jassemin and Vallée 1999.

46 Bernard Guenée has argued that Charles VI's madness cemented the administrative powers of the government, which was forced to find a way to represent the king's majesty without the king himself. He notes that '[l]a maladie de Charles VI a appris au royaume à vivre, ou plutôt à survivre, tant bien que mal, sans le roi, en exultant la royauté'. Guenée 2004, p. 262.

charnels, which can be translated as their 'relatives and immediate family', according to Claude Gauvard's examination of the terms.[47] Even in those cases where criminals seeking remission claimed to have been mad at the time of the act but sane when applying for the king's mercy, they used the language of madness to emphasize the difference between their 'normal' behavior and their behavior while out of their senses. Letters for the mad, then, were at a rhetorical level even further removed from the event they purported to describe than the majority of remission letters, which were written from the perspective of the sane criminal.

II. Languages of Madness from Families and Notaries

Most remission letters give no clear indication of the social status of the remission seekers, but those that do exhibit a broad social range, from beggars and manual laborers to merchants and nobles.[48] Many of those identified in the letters according to profession were skilled artisans, including butchers, bakers, barrel makers, and carpenters. The majority of supplicants were identified simply as laborers, often 'poor' laborers. With some exceptions, it is unlikely that these remission seekers would have been educated, and very few would even have been literate in French. The supplicants would have been familiar with a number of methods of constructing a narrative, however. The tradition of storytelling, the requirement of yearly confession, and the sermons and saints' lives read to them by their priests all provided exempla for creating a coherent tale.

In contrast, the notaries who wrote the letters down and helped compose them were not only literate but Latinate.[49] Since the royal notaries were often trained in law and remission letters were part of the greater legal system in France, legal questions were central to their construction.[50]

47 Gauvard 1991, vol. 2, pp. 643–651.

48 43% of the letters provide some indication of status, and these are randomly scattered throughout the 150 year period covered by this study, with no suggestion of change over time in terms of the frequency with which social status was mentioned nor in terms of the status of remission seekers.

49 Many were university-trained, and some were canons before their career in the royal chancery. Information about the careers of fifty-one royal secretaries and twenty-four royal notaries under Charles VI, fifteen of whom overlap, can be found in the online database, 'Opération Charles VI,' (Laboratoire de Médiévistique occidentale de Paris). Ten out of the sixty men listed were canons, and many of these held multiple ecclesiastical positions.

50 Mireille Desjardins, in a discussion of royal notaries in the fifteenth century, notes that 'Outre la langue et l'écriture latine et française, ils doivent connaître les droits coutumiers et romain,

Some notaries were officially *licencie en lois* ('licensed in law'), many were ennobled by the king for their service as royal notaries, and a few rank among the famous French humanists of the fourteenth and fifteenth centuries, including Gontier Col and Jean de Montreuil, famous for their debate with Christine de Pizan on the subject of the *Roman de la Rose*.[51] Often the positions were passed down from father to son or through other family connections, as genealogical studies of the notaries from later periods show.[52] Jean de Rinel, who helped compose Jehannecte Troppé's letter, was the nephew by marriage of Pierre Cauchon, Bishop of Beauvais, who was also chaplain to the Duke of Burgundy. Jean's position as a royal notary for the English court in France was gained partly through the Bishop's influence, and he acted as scribe in 1429, when his uncle-in-law prosecuted Joan of Arc.[53] In addition to their work in the royal chancery, the fifteenth century saw a particularly important flowering of notarial writing in literary and political arenas, and Jean de Rinel was involved in this extension of notarial works. His most significant work in this arena was his 1435 treatise defending the Treaty of Troyes against those who claimed that Charles VI's madness invalidated it.[54] Jean de Rinel, then,

les ordonnances royales et la jurisprudence qui s'appliquent au royaume afin de comprendre les consequences légales des documents qu'ils rédigent'. Desjardins 1997, p. 88. See also Lapeyre and Scheurer 1978.

51 See Gauvard 1997, p. 288. For the documents from the debate between these notaries and Christine de Pizan, see McWebb 2006.

52 Unfortunately, the most extensive studies of the identities of the royal notaries begin in the reign of Louis XI in 1461, towards the end of the period studied here. See Lapeyre and Scheurer 1978.

53 At Joan's trial, where Jean de Rinel acted as notary, there was no attempt made to explain Joan's visions in natural terms. Her accusers ignored the theoretical framework provided by medical treatises. Her visions, they claimed, 'proceeded from lying, evil spirits, rather than from good; and everyone should treat them as such, especially considering her cruelty, pride, haughtiness, actions, lies, and contradictions'. The full focus of the theological attack on Joan centered around her pact with the devil. Unlike Jehannecte Troppé, whose family could slide easily between one explanatory frame and another, Joan of Arc's accusers found it necessary to establish only one truth, since their case against her rested on proving she was demonically, not divinely, inspired. Hobbins 2005, 125–138. Pierre Champion included a brief biographical sketch of Jean de Rinel in his edition of Joan of Arc's trial, Champion 1920–1921, p. 338.

54 In 1435, Jean de Rinel wrote a treatise defending the Treaty of Troyes, in which he concentrated on the natural effects of King Charles VI's madness. Chaplais 1982, pp. 650–651. Many notaries composed political treatises as part of their work in the chancery, most of which, as Craig Taylor argues persuasively, were intended to be distributed to each other for facilitating diplomatic missions and the creation of new treaties. Particularly as Charles VII's campaign grew more successful in the 1430s, notaries worked to prove that the Treaty of Troyes was not legally sound,

can act as a particularly adept guide through the complex relationships that royal notaries had with the concept of madness. Bearing in mind that these letters were carefully constructed by a group of composers, and the resulting narrative had to be acceptable to all parties involved, how did the notaries and the family members work together to tell these stories? Only a small percentage of the letters mention madness (one percent of the total), but these provide compelling evidence for the ways in which it was defined and interpreted.

Faced with the task of explaining Jehannecte Troppé's murder of her husband, Jean de Rinel coordinated with her family to find a way of narrating the story that focused on her aberrant behavior leading up to the moment of the crime. The letter deployed multiple terms to establish that behavior as caused by mental imbalance. According to Jehannecte Troppé's letter, in October, more than two weeks before she killed her husband, Jehannecte had begun seeing visions that made her believe her husband had left her alone at night and caused her to become 'merencolie'. The next day, she acted as if she were 'demoniacle', and her husband recognized that her actions came from 'frenaisie et merencolie', or possibly from 'mal du saint',[55] and did not punish her for them, hoping that soon she would return to her 'bon sens et advis'. Unfortunately, she did not, and on the fateful night when she killed her husband, she again saw a 'vision' and 'par temptacion mauvaise de l'ennemi' she beat him with a rock. Afterwards, 'non sachant qu'elle faisoit ou disoit' she did not run away but rather stayed with her spouse without understanding that she was guilty of injuring him. Her relatives indicated that she was still, two months later, 'comme demoniacle', and due to her 'maladie' should not be punished for her crime, adding that she should be released from prison, not only for her own health but for the health of the

focusing on the mental state of Charles VI as part of their arguments. As Craig Taylor argues, the polemical works generally appear in very few manuscripts and contain cross-references to treaties contained in the chancery archives in an effort to aid those notaries and secretaries of the king sent on diplomatic missions. Taylor 2000, p. 216. In this he is mostly arguing against scholars like P.S. Lewis, who insist on reading these treatises as propaganda pieces intended for a wider audience. Lewis 1965, p. 217. Jean de Rinel had been part of the delegation sent to negotiate the Treaty of Troyes in 1420, and was probably the notary assigned to copy the text, since his name was attached to it, thus giving him an intimate knowledge of the text itself as well as of the negotiations leading up to it. For more on his relationship to Pierre Cauchon and his participation in the Treaty of Troyes, see Neveux 1987, p. 70. Neveux also includes a genealogy for Cauchon, which lists Jean de Rinel's children and their professions, including one canon and a greffier (following in his father's footsteps).

55 'Mal du saint' could be understood as an illness visited on someone as punishment for offending a saint. See Briggs 1989, p. 24.

child she was carrying. Finally, they cited the customary laws of Normandy, asserting that, if released from prison, Jehannecte would be kept in chains or otherwise securely guarded so that she would not harm anyone else in future.[56]

The religious, literary and political spheres in which the notaries interacted with each other and with other intellectuals may not have often had a direct impact on their work in the royal chancery, but in a case like Jehannecte Troppé's, Jean de Rinel was able to bring to bear his own knowledge about different types of visionary experiences in offering a possible vocabulary for her family's letter. The story they constructed reveals the variety of terms available in French to describe a mental disturbance that could lead to violence. The range of words and phrases used in describing Jehannecte Troppé suggest some of the complexities and confusions involved in describing an internal state that could be recognized through behavioral signs. The composers of Jehannecte Troppé's letter of remission, like many others writing on behalf of people whose actions had been interpreted as mad, included a number of different terms to describe her behavior. Wendy Turner and Irina Metzler have both attempted to create taxonomies of terms for madness in medieval texts.[57] While the sources they focus on support such rigid lines between definitions, the composers of remission letters rather seem to pick from a grab bag of possible terms without worrying too much about the kinds of careful distinctions made in more theoretical discourses. There are certainly continuities across the discourses that addressed madness, and some of this common ground was reflected in the understanding of madness in these letters. Although the use of these terms suggests an awareness of wider discourses about madness and its meanings, the letters seldom fully engaged with any of these larger conceptual frameworks. Particularly because these letters were not dependent upon any single discourse, they can be used in aggregate to establish a lexicon of madness.[58]

56 AN JJ 173 fo 33v no 63. Edited in Le Cacheux 1907–1908, vol. 1, pp. 181–183: 'melancholy'; 'demonically possessed'; 'frenzy and melancholy'; 'illness of the saint'; 'good sense and vision'; 'vision'; 'by evil temptation of the enemy [Satan]'; 'not knowing what she did or said'; 'as if possessed by a demon'; 'illness'. The customary law of Normandy does call for the chaining or guarding of the mad to prevent their harming themselves or others. Gruchy 1881, p. 184 LXXIX. See my discussion of the law codes below, in Pfau 2010b, and in Pfau 2008, chapter 3.

57 Turner 2013b; Turner 2013a, pp. 17–29 and p. 69; Metzler 2016, pp. 31–52.

58 For an important list of terminology used in English sources, see Turner 2013a Appendix I, pp. 233–238.

Table 1 Terms

Terms	Number of letters	Total Frequency	Terms	Number of letters	Total Frequency
Sens	70	84	Lunatique	5	5
Fol	51	53	Cognoissance	5	5
Malade	32	32	Raison	4	4
Fureur	29	34	Enragie	2	2
Entendement	28	29	Altere	2	2
Frenaisie	19	19	Aliene	2	2
Memoire	18	18	Caduque	2	2
Simple	15	15	Sot	2	2
Idiot	12	12	Cervel	2	2
Melancholie	11	11	Estonne	2	2
Savoir	10	10	Affoible	1	1
Forsene	8	14	Fatuite	1	1
Desespere	8	8	Esmouvance	1	1
Estourdi	6	6	Insane	1	1
Ignorance	6	6	Teste	1	1
Demoniacle	5	5	Dyable	1	1
			demens captui	1	1

Note that the total number of letters examined is 155.

There are two main types of language that composers of remission letters for mad people used. There was the negative language implying a loss of some cognitive ability, or the more complicated idea of being 'outside' it. Most often the loss or externality referred to the 'sense', 'understanding', 'memory', or 'knowledge'. The composers could also choose from a wide range of adjectives or nouns, each of which was recognizably part of a discourse of madness, including 'frenzied', 'furious', 'melancholic', 'demoniac', and 'foolish' (see Table 1). On average, the letters used two completely different terms, but some letters had as many as seven, suggesting that the composers were aware of the range of terminology available to describe what they perceived as mad behavior. The terms *sens*, *fol*, *fureur*, and *entendement* were sometimes involved repeatedly in a single letter, perhaps indicating that they were particularly resonant words. In their attempts to find a conceptual vocabulary about madness, the composers of remission letters had a number of different cultural resources from which to draw. The language used to describe madness in remission letters varied widely. The composers drew from many of the available discourses, creating a fluid vision of what madness was. Through a process of collaboration, the mad person's family members told their story to the royal notary, who translated it into a framework that would make sense to the family, the king's council, and ultimately the adverse party.

Notaries and Literary Circles

Beginning in the mid-fourteenth century, Charles V supported a large-scale translation project that sought to make French an intellectual language equal to Latin. The literary debate about the *Roman de la Rose* provides a vivid snapshot of the repercussions of this effort, as well as of the larger intellectual community in which the royal notaries took part. The *Roman de la Rose* survives in over 300 manuscripts and has been called one of the most read works of the Middle Ages.[59] Certainly it was one of the most contentious. Those involved in the debate drew on an extensive knowledge of philosophy, law, theology, literature, and especially classical authors. The participants, many of whom have been seen as France's earliest humanists, included important fifteenth-century theologians from the University of Paris, such as Pierre d'Ailly and Jean Gerson; literary figures at court, particularly Christine de Pizan; and the royal notaries Jean de Montreuil and Gontier and Pierre Col.[60] Claude Gauvard, in an article about the royal notaries, notes that 'the letters signed by Gontier Col or Jean de Montreuil do not stand out from the quality of the rest. These humanists reserved their genius for epistolary relations that were less constraining!'[61] While this is certainly the case (and indeed one would not expect otherwise in terms of rhetorical exuberance), the notaries' intellectual exploits nevertheless had an impact on their knowledge of and interest in particular subjects.

Jean de Meun expanded Guillaume de Lorris's brief *Roman de la Rose* between 1270 and 1280, around forty years after the original author's death, as Jean de Meun claimed. He turned the text into a philosophical allegory, where personifications of virtues and vices sought to instruct the Foolish Lover (*Fol Amoureux*) towards his goal of capturing the Rose, symbol of a woman's maidenhead. The *Roman*'s Foolish Lover wandered through a landscape filled with allegorical figures spouting classical authorities and examples before finally possessing his Rose. Two of these figures, the

59 Guillaume de Lorris and Jean de Meun 1992, p. 5.

60 There is a vast literature on the relationships between these participants. See Combes 1973, Coville 1934. More recent work has been concerned with Christine de Pizan in addition to the men, particularly Huot 1993.

61 Gauvard 1997, 288: 'des lettres signées Gontier Col ou Jean de Montreuil ne tranchent pas sur la qualité de l'ensemble. Ces humanistes réservent leur génie à des relations épistolaires moins contraignantes'!

Jealous Husband and the Duenna, proved particularly troubling to Jean de Meun's critics. The Jealous Husband claimed that no woman was pure and cursed the whole sex, while the Duenna proved these words by offering her services as a go-between for the Lover and Fair Welcome, whom he wished to woo into giving him access to his Rose. The *Roman* raised philosophical questions of whether words were inherently bad and whether it was legitimate for an author to write from the perspective of a morally questionable person. At one moment in the text, the figure of Reason described love as a paradox: 'C'est reson toute forsenable / C'est forcenerie resnable' ('It is reason completely mad / It is madness reasonable').[62] In this formulation, the author was drawing upon two possible understandings of madness.[63] First, madness was presented as a corruption of reason, and a loss of sense or wisdom. At the same time, the text developed the Biblical inversion that will be discussed below, where folly could appear as reason and wisdom, and vice versa. Interestingly, reason appears relatively rarely in the remission letters, only being used four times, while the different variations on *forsene* appear fourteen times in eight different letters. As we shall see, this latter term was drawn from the legal discourse with which royal notaries would have been very familiar.

The response to the *Roman* began with the political question of French supremacy, since it filled the role of representative of the French language in humanist circles, much as Dante's *Divine Comedy* did for Italian. Petrarch, for example, argued that 'orators and poets were not to be sought outside of Italy'.[64] In this sense, then, the defense of the *Roman de la Rose* was an integral part of the larger project of promoting French as an intellectual language in which philosophical concepts could be expressed and explored. In 1401, Christine de Pizan shifted attention to women's social and political roles, a particularly potent area of debate at a time when the Hundred Years War made Salic Law central to Valois legitimacy.[65] The debate about language, focused both on the relationship between signifier and signified

62 Guillaume de Lorris and Jean de Meun 1992, p. 282, ll. 4296–4297 and l. 4320.

63 *Forsené* was also used in other medieval literary texts. Tobler and Lommatzsch 1925–, vol. 3, pt. 2, pp. 2146–2149.

64 Petrarch, *Seniles* 9.1: 'oratores et poete extra Italiam non querantur'. Quoted in McWebb 2006, p. 2.

65 After the death of Charles IV of France, there were serious questions about the succession. The French chose to invoke Salic Law, which declared the French throne could not be inherited through a woman. This meant that Edward III, the English King and son of Isabella (daughter of the Capetian French King), was not a legitimate heir to the French throne, and the Valois cadet branch was instead. This was one of the key factors that led to Edward's war against the French that developed into the Hundred Years War.

and the question of voice (in other words, whether a moral person should write immoral things if they are written in the character of an immoral person), was especially pertinent in 1401, since Charles VI had passed a law making blasphemy a crime punishable by death.[66] Language mattered, and the questions of who was speaking in a text, the author or a character, and of whether a word could be morally bad of itself or whether words were naturally good and only the object could be morally bad, held philosophical weight. Indeed, this question may have seemed particularly compelling to the royal notaries, who engaged daily in the composition of narratives from the perspective of self-confessed criminals. Perhaps it is unsurprising, then, that these notaries were so firm in their defense of Jean de Meun's *Roman*.

While Jean de Montreuil and Gontier Col both wrote private letters in praise of Jean de Meun, and in response to his critics, neither chose to directly enter the public debate with Christine de Pizan, instead placing that challenge on the shoulders of Pierre Col, Gontier's brother. Jean de Montreuil sent a letter to Gontier Col in late July or early August 1401, calling upon Gontier to aid his defense of Jean de Meun and saying,

> it will be up to you as the leader, prince, and director of this undertaking to defend such a praiseworthy and beloved imitator, and to tread underfoot these sick and mad [*malesanos et deliros*] [critics] and to strengthen, arrange in order, and overlay my half-baked reasonings with the sharpness of your eloquence, inasmuch as I, relying on the confidence of your help and the wealth of your genius, have entered this battlefield, something I would otherwise not have done.[67]

Since Gontier Col was responsible for introducing Jean de Montreuil to the *Roman de la Rose*, Jean argued that he was justified in seeking his friend's aid in defending the work. The imputation of madness to the critics of the *Roman* is telling, particularly since Jean de Montreuil uses the word *delirus*, with its connection to delirious and raving madness. Although the negation

66 Stein 1908, pp. 153–154; Vilevault and Bréquigny 1763, vol. 10, p. 243.

67 'Quorum pretextu in alterum istorum patronorum scriptotenus invexi, sicut videbis per eam quam tibi fert epistolam is baiulus. Tuum ergo erit, dux, princeps rectorque huius cepti, laudatissimum et amatissimum imitatorem tuum defensare, et hos malesanos et // deliros conculcare ac ratiunculas meas indigestas disertie tue acumine validare, comere et linire, quatenus ego, qui auxilii tui confidentia ac ingenii ope fretus, campus hunc duelli introii, alias non facturus. Scio enim quod ubi obdormientes tui sensus expergiscentur, et calamus iacens excret se, 'non prevalebunt adversus nos' isti veritatis inimici, sed eos, cum voles, non dubito efficies oves mittes, et mutos reddes per omnia tanquam truncos.' McWebb 2006, pp. 208–209.

of the term *sens* was the most commonly used phrase to describe madness in remission letters, *malesanos* (the concept of bad sense) does not appear at all, nor does there appear to be a direct translation of *delirus*. Clearly these notaries were aware of and comfortable with the use of the literary and symbolic languages of madness and lovesickness. When composing letters of remission, they certainly did not display their literary abilities nor did they draw from the same vocabulary, but nevertheless, the larger intellectual communities to which they belonged influenced their concepts of narrative structure and their concerns about language.

Another active member of these humanist circles, Laurent de Premierfait, had a number of connections with the French court. He engaged in correspondence with several humanist royal notaries while he was living in Avignon at the papal court. When he moved to Paris, he worked as a clerk for one of the king's secretaries, which would have brought him into even closer contact with the royal court. Laurent de Premierfait was translating, and expanding upon, Giovanni Boccaccio's *De Casibus Illustrium Virorum* (*The Fall of Noble Men*), making it available to a French audience in the vernacular under the title *Des cas des nobles hommes et femmes*. In 1400, he translated the work directly, but in 1409 he revised the original, returning to the classical sources and expanding considerably on Boccaccio's original. When he finished his revised version, he was working as secretary to Jean, duke of Berry, uncle to King Charles VI, and patron of a number of important works of literature and art.[68]

In Laurent de Premierfait's 1409 retelling of the story of Cadmus, king of Thebes, the king's family members play a central role in his downfall.[69] The first disruptive episode in Cadmus's life involved his daughter. As Laurent told the story,

> while the women of Thebes were, according to their custom, performing the festival of Bacchus, Agane, daughter of the said Cadmus, became insane [*forsennee*] and went to the court as if enraged [*enraigee*] against her son Pantheus, whom she had had with Echion her husband, a noble and powerful man. And Agane struck and murdered her son Pantheus who had mocked the sacrifices that were done to Bacchus, the god of

68 For more on Laurent de Premierfait's life and works, see the essays collected in Bozzolo 2004.

69 This was Laurent de Premierfait's second translation of Giovanni Boccaccio's *De Casibus Virorum Illustrium* (*The Fall of Noble Men*). The story of Cadmus in both Boccaccio and Laurent de Premierfait was drawn from Euripides' play, *The Bacchae*. See Boccaccio 1962, p. 31; Euripides 2001.

> wine, and as some people say she murdered him with a javelin or a club while the said Pantheus was not thinking of anything; thus as Agane, returning to her senses [*sens*], afterward heard it told.[70]

Agane, becoming *forsennee* and *enraigee*, created ruptures within her family, and attacked those she would normally hold dear. These terms appear rarely in remission letters (*forsene* in eight and *enragie* in two). On the other hand, the concept of being outside of and returning to one's senses appears in seventy letters (forty-five percent of the total). Pantheus had mocked the sacrifices of the Bacchanal, which placed Agane's act in the context of a challenge to her religious community. While in ordinary circumstances Pantheus's challenge would not have led his mother to such a violent anger, the impetus of the ritual of the Bacchanal pushed her beyond her normal behavior, making her 'enraged'. The pathos of the passage is highlighted through both the emphasis on Pantheus's identity as Agane's legitimate son and Pantheus's lack of fear or concern when his mother appeared. Significantly, much like Jehannecte Troppé, Agane lost her memory of her own actions while she was 'insane', requiring others to tell her about her own deeds when she returned 'to her senses'. Her memory loss further confirmed the altered state in which she had murdered her child, and created a need for a narrative reconstruction of events that allowed Agane and her family to explain and comprehend the horror of her son's death.

Agane's actions were not the only violent episode in Cadmus's family. In a second occurrence, the husband of another of Cadmus's daughters also attacked his children.[71] Laurent explained

> Athamas, son-in-law of Cadmus, who was already called king of Thebes and to whom the people did honor as if he were already king, became enraged [*enraigié*] and crazy [*sot*], to such an extent that Athamas, believing that his wife Ynoe, daughter of the said Cadmus, was a lioness and that

70 Gathercole 1968, pp. 123–124: 'tandiz que les femmes de Thebes faisoient selon leur coustume les festes de Bachus, Agane fille du dit Cadmus devint forsennee et s'en vint le cours comme enraigee contre son filz Pantheus lequel elle avoit eu de Echion son mari, noble et puissant homme. Et Agane frapa et murtry son filz Pantheus qui se moquoit des sacrifices que l'en faisoit a Bachus, le dieu du vin, et comme aucuns dient elle le murtri d'un javelot ou d'une massue tandiz que le dit Pantheus pensoit en riens, ainsi comme Agane retournee en son sens oy aprés racompter'.

71 This story was drawn from Ovid's *Metamorphoses*. See Ovid 2004, pp. 140–146. Note that, although madness ran in the family here, it was not attributed to heredity, since Agane and Athamas were not related by blood, only by marriage.

> his two small children were two lions, gave a great cry. And afterwards, by force, he grabbed Learcus, their son together, out of the arms of Ynoe, and knocked and broke [the child] with all his effort against a hard rock. But immediately Ynoe, the mother of Learcus, upset at his death, fearing for Meleatrix, another of her sons, and fleeing Athamas, her husband, who followed her, maddened [*forseneux*] and enraged [*enraigié*]; she threw herself, with her said son Meleatrix, off the crest of a mountain into the Ionean Sea, and because of this she and her son were swallowed up and died in that sea.[72]

These two moments of violence have clear parallels, as both Agane and Athamas destroy the next generation, erasing Cadmus's lineage as well as their own. The terminology Laurent de Premierfait used to describe this madness, these mental states in which such violent actions were possible, carries over from one event to the other. Athamas, like Agane, was described as *enraigié* and *forseneux*. Their mental states were not identical: Athamas was also described as *sot*, a word that appears in only two of the remission letters related to madness (though drunkenness does appear in many other letters). Athamas' behavior manifested itself in terms of visions, rather than religious ecstasy. His visions were distinct from Jehannecte Troppé's as he saw his family transformed into wild animals rather than imagining their absence. Nevertheless, in both cases the focus was on a transformation of the normal into the frighteningly strange, both for the sufferer him- or herself and for the family members who did not expect to be the target of his or her aggression. These literary representations constructed a dichotomy between the expected behavior and the actual behavior of the subject, who destroyed communal and familial relationships by attacking the very people that he or she logically should protect.

In contrast to Laurent de Premierfait's expansion of the work, Boccaccio's treatment of Cadmus's violent and mentally unstable relatives was truncated, and used less varied and evocative language. In his Latin version, Agane was

72 Gathercole 1968, p. 124: 'Athamas, gendre de Cadmus, que l'en surnommoit ja roy de Thebes et auquel le peuple fasoit honneurs comme se il feust ja roy devint enraigié et sot, en tant que Athamas, cuidant sa femme Ynoe fille du dit Cadmus feust une leonnesse et que ses deux petis enfans feussent deux leonceaux, fist un grant cri. Et aprés par force il arracha de entre les bras de Ynoe Learcus leur commun filz, et le quoti et froissa de tout son effort contre une dure roche. Mais tandiz que Ynoe la mere de Learcus courroucee de sa mort doubtoit de Meleatrix un sien autre filz et fuyoit Athamas son mary qui la poursuivoit forseneux et enraigié, elle avec son dit filz Meleatrix se trebucha de la creste d'une montaigne en la mer Yonie, et par ainsi elle avec son filz fut transgloutie, et mourut en celle mer'.

'furiis agitata' when she killed her son, and Athamus 'in furorem lapsus'.[73] Laurent de Premierfait's translation thus moved beyond the simple image of fury, seeking multiple terms to describe Agane's and Athamas's madness. These vernacular French terms suggested particular contexts within which these moments of mental instability could be understood.

In 1409, stories about madness, kingship, family and community such as Laurent de Premierfait's would have had a particular resonance for French readers. Charles VI, the French king, had turned on his own men in 1392, in an episode his contemporaries believed was caused by a mental disturbance, and the king continued to suffer unpredictable relapses.[74] Indeed, as Nigel Mortimer has argued, citing the illustrations in the manuscript tradition, 'the *De casibus* narratives of the fallen figures of mythology, the Bible, antiquity, and recent history appear to have been used in France to comment on the political events of the present'.[75] Ducal patronage from the king's uncle widened Laurent's audience beyond his own humanist circles to the court itself, where his treatment of the madness of kings and princes would certainly have been read in the light of the potential tragedies inherent in Charles VI's own illness. Both the literary and political significance of languages of madness would have been recognized by the royal notaries, who engaged in a similar process of searching for appropriate French terminology to help them describe the condition of these remission seekers.

Medicine and Natural Philosophy

The single most common word used to indicate madness in remission letters is the negation of the word *sens*. This concept of madness as a negation of cognitive ability drew upon medieval medicine and natural philosophy. What did it mean to be *hors du sens, hors d'entendement, hors du memoire*, or all three? The medical knowledge available to the average person in the Middle Ages was not particularly complex, but it is clear from the remission

73 Boccaccio 1962, p. 31.

74 For more on the French King's madness and its representation in chronicles, see Pfau 2008, Chapter 2; Guenée 2004; Famiglietti 1986; Autrand 1986. A recent book by Julie Singer has explored the ways contemporary literary texts used the language of machines and metal to think creatively about mental health in the context of the king's madness. See Singer 2018, especially pp. 79–172.

75 Mortimer 2005, p. 34. He points out that one manuscript version includes an image of Charles VII presiding over the trial of Jean, duke of Alençon, accused of conspiracy with the English and executed.

letters that some general ideas of illness and health were shared commonly.[76] The royal notaries were not likely to be trained in medicine, but their understandings of the body would have been more informed by medical theory than those of the people seeking remission. Certainly, they would have been aware of the medical terms available to speak about madness. As part of the emerging professional classes, the royal notaries had a number of links to physicians in the late Middle Ages. For example, Christine de Pizan was the daughter of a royal physician and the wife of a royal notary. These kinds of marriage ties were not unusual, but perhaps more significantly for the question of language, several royal notaries owned medical texts, including some in translation. Jean de Montaigu, notary and secretary for Charles VI, owned a copy of the French translation of Bartholomaeus Anglicus's *On the Properties of Things*. In the section on the brain, the book explains the Galenic understanding of cognitive processes. This involved a tripartite model of the brain, where imagination (*ymaginacion*) was in the warm and dry front, reason (*raison*) in the warm and moist middle, and memory (*memoire*) in the cold and dry back.[77] Thus, the areas of the brain also correspond to three of the four humors (only phlegm is left out), with imagination associated with choler, reason associated with blood (a sanguine nature), and memory associated with melancholy.[78]

Isidore of Seville, in his sixth-century *Etymologies*, used the tripartite model of the brain to provide a model of mental illness under the heading of Chronic Diseases, dividing the general category of madness into three specific types: epilepsy, mania, and melancholy, which arise from imagination, memory, and reason, respectively.[79] Bartholomeus Anglicus followed this same effort to tie types of madness to different areas of the brain, but for him, mania (*manie*), otherwise known in medical discourse as *amance*, was an injury to the imagination, melancholy (*melancolie*) was an injury to the reason, and lethargy (*litargie*) was an injury to the memory.[80] Regardless of which illness was linked with which part of the brain, this division allowed for a more complicated reading of behavior to explain disturbances believed

76 Pouchelle examines Henri de Mondeville's fourteenth-century *Chirurgie* as a central piece from which to extrapolate about the metaphorical world of the body in the Middle Ages. See especially her discussion of methodology, Pouchelle 1990, pp. 95–100.

77 British Library (henceforth abbreviated as BL) Additional 11612 fo 53v. See also Harvey 1975, p. 35; Klibansky, Panofsky, and Saxl 1964, pp. 68–69.

78 Wendy Turner has a helpful exploration of the location of different types of mental illness in the brain. See Turner 2013a, pp. 66–76.

79 Isidore of Seville 1911, IV.7; Isidore of Seville 2006, p. 111.

80 BL Additional 11612 fo 104v.

to be caused by madness. Problems with the imagination generally produced visions, problems with the memory caused forgetfulness, and problems with the reason caused people to do irrational things.[81]

According to humoral theory, madness, like any other disease, was caused by an imbalance of the humors, but particularly an extreme excess of any one of them. Thus, madness could result from an increasingly serious case of another disease. In this sense, the illness was understood to be physiological. Although madness was concentrated in the brain, where they believed the mind was located, physicians also saw it as a disease that affected the entire body of the individual. One common perceived cause of madness in remission letters was illness, often a fever that made the person act in unexpected and inexplicable ways, or a blow to the head that caused temporary or permanent damage to a person's brain.[82]

A fever or other disease was often mentioned as the source of a temporary madness that led in many cases to suicide.[83] Interestingly, illness could even be seen as a legitimate catalyst for suicide without the addition of madness, as it was in the case of Jehan du Puy, who was purportedly on his deathbed due to illness in 1420. He had made his will, confessed, and received extreme unction before cutting his own throat. The composers of his letter explained his actions by suggesting he committed suicide because of 'temptation of the enemy, because of the oppression of his illness, or from some other cause',[84] but they did not suggest madness as an excuse. Other letters, in contrast, focused particularly on the ways in which illness could lead to a frenetic or melancholic state that made the person in question no longer responsible for any action.

The mental repercussions of being hit on the head were well understood in the Middle Ages, and in fact often the temporary results of being *estourdie*, or 'stunned', were used as an explanation for questionable actions in tavern brawls.[85] It was also understood that getting hit over the head hard enough could cause lasting damage, as was the case for Guillaume Audoyn, who

81 Klibansky, Panofsky, and Saxl 1964, p. 93. See also the chart of the Aristotelian division of souls in Park 1988, p. 466.

82 This is also apparently true in records of medieval English law courts dealing with criminal cases. Butler 2015, pp. 199–200.

83 Thirty of the one hundred forty-five letters examined mention a 'maladie', either as the original source of the madness or as an integral part of the madness.

84 AN JJ 171 fo 94v no 156: 'pour ce que par temptacion de lennemj pour cause de loppression de maladie ou autrement il sest coppes la gorge en commectant homicide de lui mesme'.

85 See the references to becoming 'estourdie' after a blow to the head in AN JJ 220 fo 227v no 380 (in 1489); AN JJ 209 fo 55 no 93 (in 1480); AN JJ 199 fo 317v no 502 (in 1465); AN JJ 131 fo 39v no 69 (in 1387); AN JJ 172 fo 113v no 221 (in 1422); and AN JJ 173 fo 250v no 524 (in 1426).

had fallen off a ladder in 1403 and hit his head. Guillaume was considered 'sourt', 'insensible', and 'ydiot' for two years before anything serious occurred. Indeed, he was capable of continuing to perform manual labor, since disaster struck while he and his wife were loading manure onto a cart. He believed she was mocking him with her movements, and 'because he was stupid and idiotic through lack of sense, angered and incensed' he knocked her over with his pitchfork and hit her several times, then drove away with the cart.[86]

Medical texts described four distinct types of madness: frenzy, mania, melancholy, and lethargy, each of which corresponded to an excess in one of the humors.[87] Avicenna's work on melancholy made it the source for all types of madness, breaking down the separation of the humors and explaining that all four humors, when burnt, could turn into melancholy. Each type of burnt humor created a particular type of madness, however, with blood creating joy and laughter, phlegm creating sloth, yellow bile creating frenzied violence, and black bile creating 'great thoughtfulness and less agitation and frenzy except when the patient is provoked and quarrels, or nourishes a hatred which he cannot forget'.[88] Of these four categories, only frenzy and melancholy appear in the remission letters.

The term *frenaisie* appeared in nineteen letters, more than any of the other types of madness described in medical texts. This term almost always appeared alongside multiple other terms, most commonly paired with *sens* or *maladie*. In fact, at times an illness was imagined as turned into a frenzy, as was the case for Denisot Sensigaut, whose 'illness of heat' caused him to 'cheu en frenoisie'.[89] Interestingly, in three letters it appears alongside *melancholie*, suggesting that the composers of remission letters were less concerned with differential diagnosis than with using terms that were

86 AN JJ 160 fo 70v no 91, edited in Guérin 1909, vol. 7, pp. 80–82: 'deaf'; 'insensible'; 'idiot'; 'pour ce qu'il estoit sourt et ydiot par non sens, yré et courroucé de ce'.

87 According to Hippocrates' *De Morbo Sacro*, which Jean-Marie Fritz argues was influential for thinking about madness in the Middle Ages, frenzy and lethargy included fever, while mania and melancholia did not. This instability, according to Fritz, made mania and, especially, melancholia the focus of medical discourse in a way that frenzy and lethargy were not. Fritz 1992, pp. 133–138. However, more recently Julie Laskaris has suggested that it was not in fact known in the Middle Ages, noting 'there is no evidence that *On the Sacred Disease* was translated into Latin, so its transmission into the medieval tradition is obviously in doubt. Its reception in the Renaissance and later seemed to center not on the rational premises it brought to medicine but, ironically, on the high degree of proper religious sentiment it proved that Hippocrates had expressed'. See Laskaris 2002, p. 60.

88 Avicenna, *Liber canonis*, quoted in Klibansky, Panofsky, and Saxl 1964, pp. 88–89.

89 AN JJ 171 fo 244v no 429, edited in Longnon 1878, pp. 19-21: 'maladie des chaleurs'; 'fall into a frenzy'.

recognizably medical. The earliest letter to combine these two terms was the one composed in 1425 for Jehannecte Troppé, described above. The second was from 1459 and was written on behalf of Jacquet Morniet, a fifty-year-old man who had been suffering from a 'maladie' and 'melencolie' that had made him 'fort frenaisieux et altere de son entendement et blecie en son cerveau' for about a year before he committed murder.[90] The letter combined multiple terms and phrases from medical discourse, explaining that the melancholy illness had injured his brain, causing him to become frenzied and altered in his understanding. Finally, there is the 1474 letter written on behalf of Jehanne, the wife of Chrestien Bolu, who after giving birth to her daughter entered into a 'melancolie' because they were too poor to support their family. This melancholy made her 'insensee' so that she decided to drown herself and her children 'en ceste fureur frenaisie et toute hors du sens et entendement'.[91] Again, the letter is drawing from a number of different medical terms without distinguishing between them.

Frenesie appears in the earliest vernacular health treatise, the thirteenth-century *Le Régime du corps* by Aldobrandino of Siena. He warns against sleeping on one's back 'por ce qu'il fait maintes maladies venir, si com apoplesie, frenesie, fantosme' ('because it makes many illnesses come, such as apoplexy, frenzy, phantasm').[92] The word appears in a number of non-medical texts as well. For example, in Gautier de Coincy's *Les Miracles de la sainte Vierge*, he lists 'li frenetiques, Li fors du sens, li enragiez' together, indicating that medical and literary vocabularies were not mutually exclusive in religious texts, and suggesting a larger pattern of cross-pollination.[93] Indeed, *frenesie* also appears in literary texts. In Adenés li Roi's *Li Roumans de Cleomadès*, he explains that torment and illness 'l'assaillirent si Que en frenesie chëi' ('assail him such that he falls into frenzy').[94] This language of 'falling into frenzy' created an image of madness as a descent. In contrast,

90 The victim in the case was Jacquet's brother's wife Jehanne, who lived in the extended household along with their parents and children. Jacquet's illness had seriously limited his participation in household tasks, and his sister-in-law began to berate him one evening for his refusal to help his mother, calling him a 'mean man' who 'is worthless'. His anger, combined with his illness, caused him to lash out against her, picking up a pestle and hitting her over the head. AN JJ 188 fo 102 no 203: 'illness'; 'melancholy'; 'very frenzied and altered in his understanding and injured in his brain'; 'ung meschant homme et quil ne valoit riens'.

91 AN JJ 195 fo 268v no 1204: 'melancholy'; 'insensible'; 'in this furor, frenzy, and completely outside her sense and understanding'.

92 Cited in Tobler and Lommatzsch 1925–, vol. 3, pt. 2, p. 2236.

93 Tobler and Lommatzsch 1925–, vol. 3, pt. 2, 2236: 'those frenetics, those outside their senses, those enraged'.

94 Cited in Tobler and Lommatzsch 1925–, vol. 3, pt. 2, 2236.

use of the term *melancholie* often involves 'fullness', suggesting a surfeit of black bile or an excess of melancholic emotions. In the late thirteenth-century romance, *Sone de Nausay*, for example, one character laments, 'Je suis sans sens, sans vaillandie, Et plains de grant melancolie' ('I am without senses, without valor, and full of great melancholy').[95] In Chrétien de Troyes' *Chevalier au lyon*, Yvain is helped out of his melancholy through the power of massage: 'Tant li froia au chaut soloil Les tanples et trestot le cors Que cel cervel li issi fors La rage et la melancolie' ('She rubbed so well in that hot sun His temples and his whole body That from his brain issued all The rage and the melancholy').[96] Again, there is a suggestion of fullness, where the melancholy and rage filled his brain and must therefore be removed in order that he return to his balanced state, and a connection between mental disturbance and emotion, as rage and melancholy were both also associated with the passions.

For the most part, this choice to use medical terms without a clear understanding of differential diagnosis is not surprising. Royal notaries were knowledgeable about the law but did not generally have medical training. However, there is a copy of Jacques Despars's commentary on Avicenna's *Canon* in the British Library that was owned by the royal notary Jean Budé, who worked for Louis XI in the late fifteenth century and was an important book collector.[97] Jacques Despars composed his commentary, which as Danielle Jacquart asserts, reads more like a collection of his own *exemplum* loosely arranged around Avicenna's work, between 1432 and 1453.[98] In book three, Avicenna discusses the signs of melancholy and includes a list of things that melancholics irrationally fear, such as the sky falling on them, the earth absorbing them, or being attacked by robbers or wolves. Jacques Despars's commentary includes a fascinating anecdote about a 'notable and famous' Parisian melancholiac (*melancholicus*) in his own time, who had an incessant fear that he would be arrested and beheaded and another about a monk who was so melancholic that he tried to throw himself out of windows.[99] While there was little effort made in remission letters to distinguish between different types of mental illness terminology, it is clear that these anecdotes about irrational fears and suicide attempts were part of common knowledge about what it meant to be mad.

95 Cited in Tobler and Lommatzsch 1925–, vol. 5, 1353.
96 Cited in Tobler and Lommatzsch 1925–, vol. 5, 1353.
97 BL Harley 4114. For more on this manuscript, see Jacquart 1980.
98 Jacquart 2001, p. 35.
99 Jacquart 1980, p. 83.

The term melancholy appears in eleven different letters, including the three discussed above. Its use spiked in the 1420s, with four of the eleven letters dating from that decade. Much like frenzy, melancholy often appears alongside other words. The most common were *sens* and *entendement*, but *malade*, *folie*, and *fureur* appeared as often as *frenaisie*. One particularly interesting letter combined seven different terms. Composed on behalf of Colin Tanquart in 1415, it described him as a young man between sixteen and eighteen who, about three years earlier, began to become diminished in his 'entendement' which made him 'furieux, ydiote, ou insensee'. More recently he had fallen into 'malencolyes par sotie et folye'.[100] The inclusion of multiple terms that, according to theoretical literature, would not be used to describe the same state, is particularly interesting here.[101] In his madness, the young Colin would paint 'fantastic' things on a large shield, then stare at them and attack the shield. According to his father, Colin continued to go to school even as his condition worsened until one night he hanged himself in the small room where he usually slept. His father found him the next morning when he went to wake him up to go to school.

Bartholomeus Anglicus's *On the Properties of Things* explained that 'the head is sometimes sick because of things that are within it, like the passions which arise in the brain such as frenzy [*frenaise*], epilepsy [*epilancie*], and their like'.[102] Bartholomeus Anglicus discusses the kinds of diseases that might affect the brain as well. He notes that the brain can retreat into itself, such that 'it does not obey as well the virtues of the soul as it appears in those who are lunatics [*lunatiques*] and in those who fall from the high illness [*hault mal*]'.[103] The 'high illness' was sometimes also referred to as *caduc* or falling sickness, which one André Guibretea suffered from in 1404, causing him to have episodes during which he became 'furieux et fol'.[104] Bartholomeus Anglicus also notes that lunatics are more troubled when the moon is new or full than at other times.

100 AN JJ 168 fo 231v no 344: 'understanding'; 'furious, idiotic, or insensible'; 'melancholy due to stupidity and folly'.

101 Irina Metzler, in particular, has established the careful categorization on the part of medieval intellectuals differentiating between what she calls congenital intellectual disability and acquired mental illness. See Metzler 2016, especially chapter 2.

102 BL Additional 11612 fo 52v: 'Le chief est aucune fois malade par cause qui est dedens lui sicomme des passions qui naissent du cervel sicomme sont frenaise epilancie et leurs sanblables'.

103 BL Additional 11612 fo 53v: 'ne obeit pas si bien ala vertu de lame si comme il appert en ceulx qui sont lunatiques et en ceulx qui chieient du hault mal'.

104 AN JJ 158 fo 168 no 360, edited in Guérin 1909, vol. 7, pp. 38–41: 'furious and foolish'.

When the brain is too dry or too moist, this causes 'the illness of small understanding [*petite dentendement*]'.[105] Bartholomeus Anglicus has a section on frenzy in which he lists a large number of French terms related to madness. He explains:

> In the 28th chapter of the book of Deuteronomy, it says that God sometimes struck people with *forsenerie* and with *folie* and with *esbahissement, forsenerie* is in this sense called *frenaisie* on which Constantine said that *frenaisie* is an aposteme that is between the skins of the brain that makes the person age and go out of his senses. And it is called *frenaisie* for the skins of the brain which are called *fresnes* as Constantine says.[106]

Here, the text uses a large number of different terms for madness, including *forsenerie*, mostly used in French legal texts, to help the reader understand the specialized medical term *frenaisie*. He also opens with a reference to the biblical text of Deuteronomy, which uses the Latin words *amentia, caecitate*, and *furore mentis* to describe the kinds of madness with which God might curse people. Though *caecitate*, as Bartholomeus Anglicus notes later in his text, translates as blindness (*avugleire*), he nevertheless explains it as a kind of blindness of reason.[107]

Law

Roman law tended to use the language of *furiosus* and *furor* to describe the kind of violent madness that might lead to criminal actions. The French vocabulary was significantly more varied, though by far the most common term used in French customary law codes was *forsené*, a translation of *furiosus*. The use of *forsené* is surprisingly rare in the remission letters; instead, they more commonly chose to use *fureur* or *furieux*. These terms were often used alongside multiple others, and indeed twice they were used together, once in 1376 and once in 1380. The letter from 1376, written on behalf of Pierre de Solente, who had murdered his nine-year-old son, used six different terms to describe his madness, explaining that he had

105 BL Additional 11612 fo 53v: 'maladie de petite dentendement'.
106 BL Additional 11612 fo 103v: 'Il est contenu ou xxvijje chapitre du livre deutronomie qui dieu fiert bat aucunes fois les personnes de forseneire et de folie et de esbahissement forseneneire est en ce propos appellee frenaisie de laquelle dit constantin que frenaisie est une apostume qui est entre les peaulx du cervel qui fait la personne veillier et yssir du sens. Et est appellee frenaisie pour les peaulx du cervel que on appelle fresnes sicomme dit constantin'.
107 BL Additional 11612 fo 104v.

become 'ydiote', 'furieux', and 'desespere' such that he had previously tried to commit suicide. He committed the act in his 'forsenerie' without 'senz ne memoire'.[108] The terms are similarly used alongside a large range of additional possible words in the 1380 case of Jehan de Moustier discussed in detail in Chapter Two. There they are used with five additional terms: 'maladie' 'insensible,' 'folie,' 'simosite,' and 'navroit memoire'. Interestingly, *forsenez* is used in the full phrase 'imbue de maligne esprit en sa dicte forsenerie', suggesting a supernatural explanation in addition to the natural one.[109]

The earliest use found for the term *forcenez* is in a blasphemy case from 1364, and it seems not to carry very much weight. The baker Jehan Razochez claims to have blasphemed because he was 'forcenez de grief' in response to the taxes he had to pay. His madness had no further effect on him, at least as recorded in the letter.[110] Later cases use the term in much more serious ways, often alongside additional language describing the madness. For example, in an infanticide case from 1379, Phote Brumel was so upset when her daughter had an illegitimate baby with their coachman, thus potentially ruining her plans for an advantageous marriage, that she became as if 'hors du sens' and threw the baby into a well 'corrociee et forsenee'.[111] Another use of the term appears in a letter that pulls from five different linguistic possibilities thrown into a single sentence. The case, also from 1379, involves Jehannecte Marchant, a young married woman guilty of theft who 'na pas bon sens naturel souvent et est merencolieuse et de forcenerie [...] par la folie' steals.[112] In a case from 1394, the term is used to describe a woman who 'comme forsenee et oultrageuse' got drunk, stayed out late, and was killed by her husband.[113] In a case from 1400, it was also used to describe a woman who had gotten drunk and was momentarily 'surprins et chargiee de vin, toute forcenee et temptee de lennemy' so that she committed suicide by strangling herself.[114] A case from 1403 recorded by the same notary describes Jehannecte de la Forge who was often 'forcenee et desmuee dentendement

108 AN JJ 110 fo 125 no 108: 'idiot'; 'furious'; 'despairing'; 'fury'; 'sense nor memory'.

109 AN JJ 118 fo 18v no 18: 'illness'; 'insensible'; 'folly'; 'stupidity'; 'has no memory'; 'filled with a malign spirit in his said fury'.

110 AN JJ 98 fo 36v no 114: 'maddened by grief'.

111 AN JJ 114 fo 116v no 236: 'outside her senses'; 'angered and maddened'.

112 AN JJ 115 fo 52 no 114: 'often does not have good, natural sense and is melancholy and from madness [...] by the folly'.

113 AN JJ 146 fo 24 no 55: 'as if mad and outrageous'.

114 AN JJ 155 fo 168 no 276: 'surprised and filled with wine, totally mad and tempted by the enemy [Satan]'.

raisonnable et de tout sens et comme forcenee et hors de sens' and cut the throat of her granddaughter.[115]

The legal landscape of late medieval France was a patchwork of competing and cooperating judicial systems. The canon law of the Church was accepted throughout France,[116] but the jurisdictions of bishops and archbishops often uneasily competed with royal justice.[117] In general terms, southern France had adopted the system of Roman law,[118] while northern

115 AN JJ 158 fo 11 no 20: 'mad and diminished in reasonable understanding and in all sense and as if mad and out of her senses'.

116 Medieval canon law crossed national borders and, theoretically at least, applied equally to all levels of society throughout Christendom, from the lowliest peasant to kings and emperors. In practice, of course, this was not the case; but, as James Brundage points out, the theory of a universally applicable law was a fascinating development even if it was not practicable. Brundage 1995, p. 3. Canon law had its foundations in the early Church, with the earliest surviving pamphlet of Church law dating from the first or second century A.D. Over time, the laws proliferated, with many decisions apparently contradicting others. In the early eleventh century, Burchard of Worms proposed that the context of each law be considered to resolve these conflicts, but it was not until Gratian's *Decretum*, composed around 1140, that an attempt was made to provide such resolutions. For a brief exploration of the history of medieval canon law, see Brundage 1995. For more detail, see Kuttner 1935 and Wintoth 2000. For more on the practice of canon law, see the essays collected in Brundage 2004. Gratian's project was an effort to synthesize the laws, providing 'an authoritative guide [...] that would permit judges and administrators to find their way through the tangled underbrush of the law with reasonable certainty and at tolerable speed'. Brundage 1995, p. 43. It presented the legal considerations dialectically, highlighting the disagreements between different decisions, but choosing one as the better alternative or determining the circumstances in which each decision had merit. As a result, Gratian's compilation became a favorite teaching text, and was thus familiar to students of law throughout Europe.

117 Nicole Gonthier has shown this in her study of Lyon. Gonthier 1993, especially pp. 19–44. This could also be true in individual cities, which were occasionally divided between the bishop's law and the local lord's law. For a rich archival study of one of these towns, see Wroe 1995.

118 Medieval knowledge of Roman law came mostly from the *Corpus iuris civilis*, which was composed of the *Institutes*, the *Digest*, the *Code*, and the *Novels*, all of which were compiled during the reign of Emperor Justinian in the sixth century A.D. The *Institutes*, produced in 533 A.D., consists of an elementary guide to Roman law, modeled after an earlier (and surviving) version dating from 160 A.D. The *Digest* was compiled between 530 and 533, and essentially gathered together the opinions of classical Roman jurists and organized them according to topics. The different jurists did not always agree with each other on each topic, but there was no attempt made on the part of the compilers to provide a single, unified response to the question under consideration. Instead, the goal of the *Digest* was to provide multiple authoritative voices addressing the same questions. Papinian, Ulpian, Modestinus, and the Laws of the Twelve Tables are the sources cited in reference to madness. The Laws of the Twelve Tables is the earliest known source for Roman private law, promulgated around 450 B.C., but only surviving in those fragments collected by later compilers. The Twelve Tables consisted of a list of legal rules, and most of what survives was concerned with family law, property, succession, and the rules for legal process. Papinian, Ulpian and Modestinus, all jurists in the third century A.D., wrote extensive commentaries on questions directed to them. These commentaries, as excerpted

France acknowledged customary law, which was regionally determined and could even vary between urban centers and the countryside. The legacy of both Roman law and canon law is evident in the compilations of French customary law when it began to be recorded in the thirteenth century. Customary law was understood as an oral tradition that drew on local memory, and as distinct from Roman and Canon law by virtue of the fact that it was not codified. As Esther Cohen argues, the myth of customary law as 'old,' 'good,' and 'pure,' specifically because of its orality, led practitioners to avoid writing down the laws until well into the thirteenth century.[119] In 1454, towards the end of the period under consideration here, the French king issued an ordinance calling for the redaction of all local customs, and when this process was completed by the middle of the sixteenth century they had been standardized to some degree, ensuring that they did not conflict with any royal ordinances. The earlier redactions of customary law, their authors often attest in their prologues, were intended to instruct those who were not knowledgeable about the law. The customals considered here are just such instruction manuals, and although a few of them were originally written in Latin, all of them have vernacular versions.[120] I have looked at the ways that

in the *Digest*, have been removed from their original context and placed next to each other. While this facilitates reference, it also makes it difficult to know whether the jurist's opinion is case-specific or intended to have wider ramifications. The compilers of the *Code*, released in 534 A.D., were specifically instructed to provide a synthesis of laws, unlike those who assembled the *Digest*, and to avoid including repetitious, contradictory, or obsolete laws. The final section of the *Corpus*, the *Novels*, comprises a collection of new laws that were created during Justinian's reign, but none of them refers to madness. For more on Roman law, see Johnston 1999, pp. 2–3, pp. 12–14, pp. 22–23.

119 See Cohen 1993, pp. 28–39.

120 See especially the prologue of Jacques d'Ableiges 1868, pp. 4–6. Many customary law books did not mention madness at all, leaving open the question about how that region legally coped with mad people. See, for one example, Marechal and Poumarede 1988. In those customals that do refer to madness, the influence of Roman law can often be detected, but they depart from Justinian's *Corpus* in significant ways. The texts under consideration for their reference to madness are mostly from the thirteenth century, although there are two later redactions as well. The earliest is the *Très-ancien Coutumier de Normandie*, found in both Latin and French manuscripts from the early thirteenth century. Tardif 1903, vol. 1. In the later thirteenth century, another version of the customs of Normandy was redacted, known as the *Ancienne Coutumes de Normandie*. Gruchy 1881. Philippe de Beaumanoir was heavily influenced by Roman law in his redaction of the *Coutumes de Beauvaisis* composed around 1283. Philippe de Beaumanoir 1970–1974, vols. 1–3; Philippe de Beaumanoir 1992. A final thirteenth century legal compilation is *Li livre de jostice et de plet* from the region of Orléans, a compilation of Roman, Canon, and some customary laws. Rapetti 1850. Jacques d'Ableiges composed his *Grand coutumier de France*, a compilation of customary law from the Île de France, at some point in the fourteenth century.

Roman and customary law addressed questions of mental competence in terms of guardianship and contractual agreements elsewhere.[121] Here, I am interested in focusing on the language used in French to describe madness in terms of crime. Following the tradition of Roman law, French customals argued that the mad should not be punished for criminal actions.

The earliest of the customals comes from Normandy and uses varied language to talk about potentially violent madness. The *Ancienne coutume de Normandie* made provisions for mad people under the heading of 'On Suicides'. Suicides were punished severely under French law. Their goods were confiscate to the crown, their bodies were often 'executed', and they would be buried in unconsecrated ground, having forfeited their right to inclusion in the community of the faithful. However, the Norman customal recommended that

> any mad [*forsené*], enraged [*enragié*], or frenetic [*frénétique*] person is not to be driven out of the community of the church, in such a case where at the time when he was well ordered in his thoughts, he carried himself as a good Christian; nor are the goods of these forfeited [to the king], if by any mischance they have been killed; but it belongs to the prelate to organize the goods of these, because they [the mad] do not have the understanding to organize them [their goods].[122]

Here the customal uses a number of different French terms to refer to madness, rather than simply using *forsené*. Both of the additional terms come from medical language and refer to a kind of active and chaotic madness. The idea that the suicide of a mad person was accidental (by 'mischance') removes any culpability, so punishment would be inappropriate if the individual in question had been 'a good Christian' while sane. This judgment parallels that of Thomas Aquinas, who determined that mad people were still able to receive baptism and the Eucharist if, when sane, they were

Jacques d'Ableiges 1868. And finally there is a mid-fifteenth-century customal from Anjou and Maine. Beautemps-Beaupré 1883, vol. 4.

121 Pfau 2010b and Pfau 2008, chapter 3.

122 Gruchy 1881, pp. 56–57, XXI: 'Et aulcun forsené, enragié, ou frénétique n'est à oster de la communie de l'Eglise, pour tant au temps qu'il estoit bien ordonné de sa pensée, il se portast bon Crestien; ne de ceulx n'est pas le chastel forfaict [au Roy], se par aucune malefortune ils ont esté occis; mais appartient au prélat à ordonner d'iceulx chastels, puisqu'ils n'ont sentement pour en ordonner'.

believers.[123] Reputation, not only as a mad person but also as a Christian, played a significant role in determining the treatment of the accused.[124]

Philippe de Beaumanoir, writing his *Coutumes de Beauvaisis* around 1283, made a distinction between the 'naturally mad', or *fous natureus*, and the 'insane', or *forsenés*, noting that 'one cannot sue on an agreement made by [...] an insane person, nor a natural mad person [...] for [...] neither an insane person nor a natural mad person [can make an agreement], because they do not know what they are doing'.[125] Although he saw these as two distinct conditions, he nevertheless discussed them under the same circumstances.[126] Philippe de Beaumanoir also suggested that neither should be punished for their crimes, but here, interestingly, he chose to use a different terminology. He suggested that if 'they commit, because of their mad senses [*fol sens*], a homicide or any other serious crime, they are not punished like others because they do not know what they are doing'.[127] Instead of being punished 'like others,' for example by being executed for committing a capital crime like homicide, Beauvaisis's customary law called for the imprisonment of the mad person after a crime was committed.

The thirteenth-century *Livres de jostice et de plet* from the region of Orléans, adds a new term to our list, one which does not appear in any of the other texts. This term, *desverie*, is used in conjunction with the usual legal term *forsené*. The text explains that, when faced with a mad person who had committed a crime,

123 Aquinas responded to the argument that the mad are like beasts and therefore should not be given the sacraments by saying that '[m]admen and imbeciles lack the use of reason accidentally, i.e. through some impediment in a bodily organ; but not like irrational animals through want of a rational soul'. Aquinas 1981, vol. 4, pp. 118–120. For the Latin, see Aquinas 1964, vol. 57, p. 120, 3a 68, 12.

124 Interestingly, the Norman customal recommended that the mad person's goods be organized by the church, since clearly a mad person would not have been capable of making a will. This opens up interesting possibilities for clashes between the officers of the crown and local prelates in suicide cases, since the crown would benefit from those found sane and the Church would benefit from those found mad, although it is not possible here to do more than speculate.

125 Philippe de Beaumanoir 1970–1974, vol. 2, ch. 34, paragraph 1061: 'L'en ne puet suir de convenance [...] forsené, ne fol naturel [...] car [...] ne li forsenés, ne li fous natureus pour ce qu'il ne sevent qu'il font'. See also vol. 1, ch. 12, paragraph 411.

126 Here I take issue with the work of Irina Metzler, who argues that the distinction between these two conditions is more significant. Metzler 2016.

127 Philippe de Beaumanoir 1970–1974, vol. 2, ch. 52, paragraph 1575: 'il font par leur fol sens aucun homicide ou aucun autre vilain cas, il ne sont pas justicié en la maniere des autres pour ce qu'il ne sevent qu'il font'.

> if you know certainly that he did it in madness [*forsenerie*], that he does not know what he does every day, and that he understands nothing, nor is there any suspicion against him, you can in a way alleviate his sentence, because he is tormented enough by his madness [*desverie*].[128]

A lack of understanding and knowledge of 'what he does every day' suggests a lack of intent and therefore of responsibility, but the jurist recommends that the sentence should be alleviated, not because of the mad person's lack of intent, but because his madness is sufficient torment. While this may be merely a rhetorical aside without much impact on the legal treatment of mad criminals, it reveals an interesting tension between the acceptance that mad people should not be held responsible for their crimes and the belief that criminal acts deserve punishment regardless of intent.[129]

Underlying the concept that mad people could not be held responsible for criminal acts was a larger philosophical tradition that determined the importance of intent. For example, in his French translation of Aristotle's *Ethics*, a copy of which was owned by the royal notary Jean de Montaigu,[130] Nicole Oresme[131] used the term *forsené* in his translation of a passage about intent, noting that 'dumb beasts who do not have any use of reason or intention or understanding, nor children or mad people [*foursenez*] who do not have the use of reason and do nothing intentionally'.[132] Though Oresme

128 Rapetti 1850, p. 73, XXI.5: 'Et se tu sés certainement que il l'ait fet en forsenerie, qu'il ne sache qu'il face toz jorz, et qu'il n'entende riens, n'en i ait point de sopeçon contre lui, tu porras en une feintise estramper sa paine, quar il est assez tormentez de sa desverie'.

129 This may in fact be related to the medieval practice of punishing animals for crimes, despite their lack of comprehension. As Jacqueline Hoareau-Dodinau points out, 'la sanction infligée par le group social à la suite d'un acte qui trouble la communauté n'est pas automatiquement liée à la notion de responsabilité au sens juridique du terme, c'est-à-dire aux notions de faute, de volonté, de liberté. Pour répondre à un crime, le groupe peut exercer une vengeance sur le coupable, écarter un danger qui le menace en éliminant l'auteur ou se purifier de la souillure résultant de l'acte sans pour autant envisager la notion de responsabilité; c'est-à-dire envisager la répression par rapport à la victime ou au groupe auquel elle appartient et non pas au égard au coupable'. Hoareau-Dodinau 2001, p. 192. See also Cohen 1993, pp. 101–133.

130 Holbrook 2006, pp. 380–381.

131 Oresme was a fourteenth-century philosopher, mathematician, and theologian commissioned by Charles V to translate a number of Aristotle's works. For a brief biography of Oresme, see Babbitt 1985, pp. 1–4. See also the brief addition to his early biography in Courtenay 2000.

132 BL Egerton 737 fo 56: 'les bestes mues qui nont point usaige de raison ne voulente ne entendement ne les enfans et foursenez qui nont pas usaige de raison ne font riens voluntairement'. For more on the philosophical development of the theory of intentionality, see the essays collected in Perler 2001.

regularly chose to translate terms related to madness by using *forsené*, he also often used the phrase *hors de bon sens*. For example, in Book 7, Chapter 5 on incontinence, the text explains that some men cannot control themselves, 'like those who sleep and those who because of an illness are out of their good sense [*na pas bien son sens*]'. Oresme also provides a glose which explains the text, saying 'some who are called *amoureux* or *amer par amours* such that they are mad and are ill from a sickness that the physicians call *amorcerois*'.[133] This terminology of lovesickness does not appear in letters of remission, but as noted above phrases like *hors de bon sens* or *na pas bien son sens* were very common.

Starting in the fourteenth century, French legal texts began to use the word *fol* to describe potentially violent madness. For example, Jacques d'Ableiges' fourteenth-century *Grand Coutumier de France* listed 'when any crime is done by any mad [*folle*] or drunken person' among a number of other reasons for altering the proscribed sentence, indicating that intent was the significant factor, since neither drunk people nor mad people are capable of intent.[134] A mid-fifteenth-century customal from Anjou and Maine also explained that 'a mad person [*fol*] who kills or mutilates a man or a woman should be kept in prison perpetually at his or her own expense. But for theft [possibly rape?] or another small crime, his or her madness excuses it'.[135] Thus, although madness could be seen as an excuse for a 'small crime', it did not excuse murder or mutilation. Even though the customal provided an alternative (and lighter) sentence for mad people, it emphasized that some form of punishment was necessary for attacking another person.

Use of the words *fou* and *folie* in letters of remission often indicated behavior similar to that described by the English terms 'fool' and 'folly'.[136] The term was only rarely used on its own, rather than in conjunction with other terms evoking madness, most often in cases of theft or rape.

133 BL Egerton 737 fo 189: 'Si comme cellui qui dort et cellui qui par la cause de maladie na pas bien son sens.' 'Si comme aucuns que lendit amoureux ou amer par amours entant quilz en afolent et sont malades dun mal que les medicins appellent amorcerois'.

134 Jacques d'Ableiges 1868, p. 649 IV.xii 'Des peines': 'quant aucun excès est faict par aucune personne folle ou yvre'.

135 Beautemps-Beaupré 1883, p. 268: 'Le fol qui occist ou mutille homme ou femme doit à ses despens estre tenu en chartre perpetuelle. Mais pour embler ou faire autre petit excès, sa folie l'en excuse'.

136 See for example AN JJ 223 no 41 fo 24v, where a drunken man is described as 'foul'; AN JJ 209 no 93 fo 55, where a drunken man uses the term 'foulx' as an insult; AN JJ 155 no 11 fo 5, where a young man steals from 'folie'; and AN JJ 155 no 309 fo 188, where young men commit gang rape through their 'folie jeunnesse'.

So, for example, a 1379 letter composed on behalf of Ysabelet de Baconne explained that she had stolen from her uncle, with whom she lived, to give to her lover because of her 'foleur' and her youth.[137] In other cases, the same terms were used as one of the array of possible terms to describe a more violent form of madness. A bar brawl in 1390 that led to murder involved Pierre Chambo 'dit le fol'. In addition to being called *fol*, the letter composed on his behalf noted that he was 'comme tout ydiote non aiant senz ne discrettion'. When he lost a great deal of money while gambling with Pierre Audrieu, called Tachat, they took their argument outside. Tachat came at Chambo with a knife, but Chambo, who had no knife or sword, killed Tachat by hitting him in the head with a stone. The composers of the letter insisted that this happened because of 'le petit sens et discrecion' of Chambo.[138] In another case that described an even more violent madness, the merchant Gile le Treulier fell into 'folie et debilitacion de son sens' because of losses and damages he had suffered. The letter also described him as 'comme furieux', all of which caused him to commit suicide in 1421.[139] *Folie*, then, could work on multiple levels of meaning, ranging from a youthful error to a serious threat to oneself or others. When it was used to describe a more serious issue, it generally appeared alongside additional terms.

The term *ydiot* was also a legal word, though it was not used in the customals to refer to the type of madness that might cause someone to commit a crime. Instead, as other scholars have shown for Europe more generally, it was used as a translation of the Latin term *idiotus* and usually referred to someone who was mad from birth.[140] It appears in twelve remission letters, however, and unlike *folie*, it is generally used alongside multiple terms to describe a kind of violent madness rather than simply foolish behavior. For example, in the earliest use found, discussed in more detail above, Pierre de Solente was described as an 'ydiote' along with five other terms when he killed his son in 1376.[141] In another case from 1391, the ironically named Jehan le Sage (who was 'given the said surname as a joke'), servant of François de L'Hospital, was 'comme idiot et lunatique'. At the instigation of a prostitute, he hit another woman and then attacked and wounded two

137 AN JJ 114 fo 142v no 270: 'folly'.

138 AN JJ 140 fo 83 no 67: 'called the fool'; 'like a complete idiot, not having sense nor discretion'; 'the little sense and discretion'.

139 AN JJ 171 fo 244v no 429: 'folly and debilitation of his sense'; 'as if furious'.

140 Turner 2013a, pp. 18-20; 28; 235–236.

141 AN JJ 110 fo 125 no 108: 'idiot'.

sergeants who responded to the scuffle.[142] While specific legal terminology was being used in remission letters, they were used far less often than other words and seldom with the kind of careful distinction between different concepts that can be seen in normative texts like law codes.

Religion

In addition to medicine and the law, religious texts also discussed mental illness. The evocative imagery of people existing outside their sense, understanding, memory, and reason stems in part from the biblical concept of the mad person, who lacks spiritual knowledge and fails to recognize God, as the opposite of the wise person. This kind of foolishness held up as the inverse of wisdom is particularly prevalent in the Old Testament and especially in the Book of Proverbs.[143] In Latin, the most common term used for this type of madness is *stultus*,[144] though perhaps the most famous reference to madness in the Psalms, *Dixit insipiens*, or 'the fool says in his heart there is no God', appears in two different Psalms.[145] Raoul de Presles translated the Bible into French as part of Charles V's translation project. In his French translation of the psalms, he translates *insipiens* as *le fol* in Psalm 13, but as 'celui qui nestoit pas sage' ('the one who is not wise') in Psalm 58.[146] This suggests that for Raoul de Presles, it was important to emphasize the way madness was the opposite of wisdom. Madness as perceived by the world was not always understood negatively in the Bible, however. Through the figure of inversion, the same terms used to describe the opposite of wise action could also be

142 AN JJ 140 fo 265 no 234: 'lui aeste le dit seurnom mis par derrision'; 'like an idiot and lunatic'. François de l'Hospital was the chamberlain of Charles VI's brother Louis, duc de Touraine at the time.

143 Several French translations of parts of the Bible were circulating in this period. Berger 1884. These stories also circulated in vernacular sermons. For more on sermons, see Zink 1976.

144 The Latin Biblical citations come from Weber 1969. See First Kings 25:25, Job 5:2, Psalms 48:11, Psalms 91:7, Proverbs 7:22, Proverbs 9:13, Proverbs 10:1–25, Proverbs 11:29, Proverbs 12:15, Proverbs 13:16–20, Proverbs 14:3–29, Proverbs 15:2–21, Proverbs 17:2–28, Proverbs 18:2–13, Proverbs 19:3–29, Proverbs 24:7–9 and 30, Proverbs 26:1–12, Proverbs 27:3 and 22, Proverbs 28:26, Proverbs 29:9–11 and 20, Proverbs 30:22 and 32, Ecclesiastes 2:12–19, Ecclesiastes 4:5, 13 and 17, Ecclesiastes 6:8, Ecclesiastes 7:5–11, 18 and 26, Ecclesiastes 10:1–6, 13–15, Ecclesiastes 18:18, Ecclesiastes 21:22 and 26–28, Ecclesiastes 22:9–22, Ecclesiastes 27:12, Isaias 32:4–6, Jeremias 10:14, Luke 12:20, and First Corinthians 3:18–19.

145 *Insipiens* gets used both in terms of folly and in terms of insanity, as these concepts are used in the Bible. See Psalm 13:1, Psalm 38:9, Psalm 52:1, Proverbs 10:18, Proverbs 14:1, Proverbs 26:8, Ecclesiastes 10:12, Ecclesiastes 20:14 and 33, and Isaias 32:5 for *insipiens* as the inverse of *sapiens*. See Psalm 48:11 and 13, Psalm 91:7, Luke 6:11, 2 Peter 2:16 for *insipiens* as insanity.

146 BL Lansdowne 1175. See also Bonnardot 1884, p. 41, p. 117, p. 143, p. 153, and p. 262.

understood as the positive state of soothsayers and prophets,[147] or the way Jesus was perceived by unbelievers.[148] One pertinent example of this comes from the Fourth Book of Kings 9:11, when the prophet Eliseus anoints Jehu. The servants present ask, 'why came this mad man to thee', referencing Eliseus. In Latin, the term is *insanus*, which Raoul de Presles translates somewhat awkwardly as 'ce hors du sens', or 'this one out of his senses'.[149] In Christian understanding, then, these terms had multiple and varied significations. In interpreting these Biblical cases and trying to understand their significance in more general terms, medieval theological texts treated madness as a loss of human reason, and Latin theological terms for madness taken from the Bible, such as *insipiens, insania,* and *dementia*, imply this lack.[150] The Latin biblical terminology for a more violent kind of madness uses the terms *insania, furor, amentia*, and *dementia* as well as occasionally *insipiens*.[151] Deuteronomy 28:28, for example, reads 'percutiat te Dominus amentia et caecitate ac furore mentis' ('the Lord strike thee with madness and blindness and fury of mind').[152] Despite the availability of French terms such as *fureur* or *enragie* to describe this type of madness, Raoul de Presles again chose to translate this concept as 'hors du sens'.[153] This was not because he did not have a sense of the alternative vocabulary, however. In Fourth Kings 19, he translates *insanus*, the same term from Fourth Kings 9, as 'forsenerie', saying that punishment comes from your 'forsenerie' against God, and that you are 'forsenez' against Him, interestingly turning to the legal terminology.

While not many of the terms used in these texts were unique to religious discourse, the term *demoniacle* indicated the involvement of a demon. This term appeared in remission letters only five times, usually with the caveat *comme* or 'as if'. In the case of Jehannecte Troppé discussed above,

147 Fourth Book of Kings 9:11 and 19:28 (*insanus*); Prophecy of Isaias 44:25 (*furor*).

148 Gospel of Mark 3:21 (*furor*); Gospel of John 10:20 (*insanus*); Acts of the Apostles 12:15 and 26:24 (*insanus*); First Corinthians 14:23 (*insanus*).

149 All English translations of the Bible come from Challoner 1971. The idea that a fool in the world could be wise in the eyes of God was picked up by a number of medieval saints, most notably St. Francis of Assisi. Saward 1980, pp. 84–89.

150 Fritz 1992, p. 7.

151 Deuteronomy 28:28 (*amentia* and *furore mentis*); Prophecy of Isaias 24:6 (*insanie*); Prophecy of Jeremias 25:16 (*insanie*); Prophecy of Zacharias 12:4 (*amentia*) Book of Wisdom 14:21–31 (*insaniae*) Gospel of Luke 6:11 (*inspientia*). In the French translation of the psalms, *furor* was translated as *fureur, insensate* as *insensible*, and *fatuus* as *fatuite*. See Bonnardot 1884, p. 41, p. 117, p. 143, p. 153, and p. 262.

152 Deuteronomy 28:28.

153 See Tobler and Lommatzsch 1925–, vol. 3, pt. 2, p. 2360. So, for example, in Brunetto Latini's thirteenth-century *Li Livres dou tresor*, he notes that 'l'om(e), quant il met son cors en peril par ire et par furor, il n'est mie fors; mais cil qui se met en peril par droite conoissance, est fors'.

for example, Jean de Rinel and her family used it to be inconclusive about whether her visions were caused by supernatural or natural sources. Both these possibilities were equally reasonable according to different strands in intellectual thought. In addition to Jehannecte Troppé's case, it is used in a 1381 letter on behalf of Denisot Bornigon, who claimed to have been falsely accused by a man who had been 'hors du sens et demoniacle' for two years and had even been taken to a saint's shrine to seek treatment.[154] Another case from 1393 involves a man who slandered the King of France, Charles VI, but who is described as 'frenetique et demoniacle' in addition to being drunk at the time of his treasonous statement.[155] In a letter from 1488, the term was used to describe a woman whose madness had been caused by a sorcerer.[156] Finally, in a case with close parallels to Jehannecte Troppé's, in 1492 Charlotte Caignaude explained that her second husband, Anthonie Fornier, drank too much and abused her so much that she would have died if the neighbors had not intervened. When she moved out of their home and went to stay with her family, Anthonie threw her belongings into the street like 'ung foul et demoniacle'.[157] In every case, the term is used in conjunction with others.

Religious ideas about the mad revolved around medieval anxieties about the relationship between body and soul, and in the fourteenth century these anxieties began to focus on the question of possession. The body ungoverned by the mind was a threat to the immortal soul, but it could also be a sign of possession, either divine or demonic. Perhaps the most disquieting aspect of madness for both theologians and physicians was that it often had no evident somatic symptoms.[158] As Jean-Claude Schmitt argues, 'demoniacs are masters neither of their desire nor of their gestures'.[159] This troubling supernatural state mirrored a state of mental disturbance. Most manifestations of madness were only recognizable through the behavior of the individual suffering from the disease, which meant that, like possession which resembled madness, it had to be discerned from externally observable behavior.[160] The instability of madness as a disease was a serious concern

154 AN JJ 120 fo 17 no 24: 'out of his senses and demonically possessed'.

155 AN JJ 144 fo 270 no 469: 'frenetic and demonically possessed'.

156 AN JJ 220 fo 6v no 12.

157 AN JJ 223 fo 24v no 41: 'a fool and demonically possessed'.

158 Fritz 1992, pp. 133–138. While frenzy and lethargy both included fever, mania and melancholia did not. This instability, according to Fritz, made mania and (especially) melancholia the focus of medical discourse in a way that frenzy and lethargy were not.

159 Schmitt 1990, p. 127: 'les démoniaques ne sont maîtres ni de leur volonté ni de leurs gestes'.

160 Nancy Caciola has done quite a bit of work on the attempts to discern possession. Although she refers to the fact that madness was a possible interpretation of possessed behavior, she does not discuss the ramifications of this possibility in detail. Caciola 2003.

for medieval theologians, because the question of whether the behavior perceived as mad was caused by a natural illness, demonic possession, or divine possession determined the treatment of the person involved.

In Nicole Oresme's *De causis mirabilium*, a work seeking natural and reasoned explanations for miraculous phenomena composed in the 1340s, before his larger project of Aristotelian translation,[161] he explained madness in relative terms, noting that everyone is affected by 'vapours in the brain'. He notes that 'certain healthy people [...] speak spontaneously and sometimes say certain things to which they are not paying attention and about which they are not thinking, like excited, angry men perhaps about wars'. Similarly, he notes that 'lighthearted people sing' without thinking about what they are doing. From this, he turns to the idea that these same vapours are involved in the behavior of maniacs and melancholics, who therefore 'are not able to be silent [...], and just as species of the fantasia occur to them, they express them so, because they do not know how to control themselves or how to hold back from what should not be said. Look inside yourself: if you were saying all the things which occur to you now on this, now on that, then no matter what or how much you said, people would surely call you a fool'.[162] Oresme defined madness, then, as an inability to censor oneself, a lack of control between thought and speech, and as springing from natural causes, these 'vapours' that arise in the brain.[163] The theory that mad people were simply saying and doing things that sane people prevented themselves from doing, not that they were saying and doing things that were completely inexplicable, creates an image of madness that is not far removed from sanity. There is indeed a method in the kind of madness Oresme imagined, even though it would be difficult for a sane person to follow the peregrinations of the

161 Bert Hansen provides an overview of Oresme's work criticizing astrology and the belief in magic. See Hansen 1985, pp. 3–16.

162 Hansen 1985, p. 252–253, III.7: 'Dico 7° quod in multis hominibus fiunt multe cogitationes et elevationes fumorum et motus in cerebro et circa instrumenta potentiarum anime et etiam sensuum exteriorum. Unde quosdam sanos videmus qui per se loquuntur et quandoque aliqua loquuntur ad que non advertunt nec de quibus cogitant, sicut animosi et irati forte de bellis aut et cetera. Et lascivi cantant in laborando quandoque et faciendo alia ita quod quamvis ad cantum suum non advertant et cetera. Et in maniacis et melancolicis ascendunt fumi multi et precipue circa cerebrum et instrumenta anime et potentiarum eius, ut notum est; ideo non possunt tacere nec etiam quiescere in aliis membris et sicut occurrunt species fantasie sic exprimunt quia nesciunt se corrigere nec abstinere a non dicendis. Vide in te: si loquereris omnia que tibi occurrunt modo de uno modo de alio, que et quot tu diceres, certe homines dicerent te fatuum'.

163 To give just one example, in AN JJ 144 no 469 fo 270, a man explains that he committed treason by calling the king mad because he himself was a 'povre homme insensible, homme frénétique et démoniacle'.

conversation. But, he suggests, it would be no more difficult to understand a mad person's conversation than to understand the random and varied thoughts of a sane person. Rather than lacking reason, Oresme suggested that mad people were merely uncensored.

Oresme went on to address the issue of the similarities between the perceived behavior of mad people and that of people possessed by the devil, arguing that, 'As to the second question [i.e. whether maniacs are demoniacs], as I have said above, those who do not know direct, natural causes flee to demons; some flee to the heavens, others to God [as the cause]. And as such things seem marvelous, people then attribute etc., but this is wrong'.[164] Oresme proceeded to explain that, since Avicenna had provided medical cures for madness, madness was clearly a physiological disease, and not a supernatural one.

Although there was a clear medical understanding of the sources of visionary experiences, at the same time that Jean de Rinel was writing on Jehannecte Troppé's behalf, the issue of discernment of spirits was becoming more and more important to theologians such as Jean Gerson.[165] Gerson focused on the similarities between somatic madness and possession, both divine and demonic. His main concern was discerning between divine and demonic possession,[166] but within this literature he also discussed the differences and similarities of possession and madness. Gerson was concerned about determining the truth of revelations, explaining in a treatise written in 1402 that, although some revelations are true, many of them come from the illness of madness, saying '[s]uch a person should think of such matters as resulting from an injury done to the imagination and should worry about being ill in the way that insane, manic, or depressive people are'.[167] Much of what

164 Hansen 1985, pp. 262–263: 'Ad aliud ut superius dixi illi qui nesciunt causas immediatas et naturales fugiunt ad demones, alii ad celum, alii ad Deum. Et quia talia videntur mirabilia ideo attribuunt et cetera, sed hoc est falsum'.

165 Indeed, as Hansen points out, Gerson was influenced by Nicole Oresme's work in his own consideration of miracles and magic. In contrast to Oresme, Gerson allowed a much larger space for demons, but he also acknowledged the possibility of natural explanations. Hansen 1985, pp. 114–119.

166 Both Caciola 2003 and Newman 1998 provide excellent, but very different, examinations of efforts to discern between divine and demonic possession. However, although both note that the behaviors exhibited by the possessed were similar to those exhibited by the mad, both authors focus more on what that means for the concept of possession, treating madness as a known entity.

167 Translation comes from Gerson 1998, p. 339. 'Et si quae talia praeter solitum evenire circa eum contigerit, rejiciat a se cum sancto, humili verecundoque pudore. Deputet talia vel laesioni

worried theologians about madness involved the popular belief that mad people had prophetic powers.

Gerson also sought to limit the excessive fasting that many female mystics were practicing.[168] Although he often mentioned the possibility that actions that might appear holy could be inspired by the devil, he also noted the likelihood that they were signs of mental disturbance. The linkage Gerson perceived between madness and fasting was actually cyclical. He explained that

> excessive abstinence and drunken overeating both lead to a similar end, except that excessive abstinence is harder to remedy, for it brings incurable illness from brain damage and mental disorder. It happens then through mania or rage or other melancholy passions that phantasms become so deeply rooted and buried in the brain that they are thought to be true objects that appear outside the mind [...] Medical books are full of such monstrous apparitions and disturbances in the power of judgment resulting from injury to the interior powers. Concerning such people, Jerome says that they are more in need of the remedies of Hippocrates than the counsel of others.[169]

The dangers of excessive fasting, according to Gerson, are physiological. By starving oneself, one can actually cause mania, rage, or melancholy to such an extent that visions occur. Gerson was willing to pass such worrisome cases on to physicians, arguing that confessors (such as himself) were not equipped to provide remedies for the physiologically insane.

propriae phantasiae, et se habere aliquid simile phreneticis, et maniacis aut melancholicis reformidet'. Gerson 1962, vol. 3, p. 40.

168 The seminal work on this topic is of course Bynum 1987. However, it is important to note the contribution to this concept by Caciola 2003. Caciola argues that Bynum and others have overemphasized the hagiographical views of the confessors who wrote these women's lives. She contends that any examination of these women's actions has to take into account the fact that they were seldom sanctioned by the church, and that the larger population viewed them with serious suspicion.

169 Gerson 1998, pp. 345–346. 'Itaque ad par exitium vergunt abstinentia nimia et crapulosa voracitas; nisi quod irremediabilior est excessus in abstinentia; quia morbos affert incurabiles ex laesione cerebri et rationis perturbatione, quo fit ut per maniam aut furiam vel caeteras passiones melancolicas sic profundantur et intime radicantur phantasmata interius reservata in cerebro, quod esse reputantur verae res extrinsecus apparentes, et audire se putat homo, videre vel tangere quod nullo modo sensu exteriori percipitur. [...] Pleni sunt medicorum libri de portentuosis hujusmodi apparitionibus et judicorum corruptionibus ex laesione virium interiorum nascentibus. De his ait Hieronymus quod magis indigent fomento Hypocratis quam aliorum consilio'. Gerson 1962, vol. 3, p. 44.

Gerson imagined the devil as the instigator of possessed behavior, but in the fifteenth century more and more focus was placed on sorcerers as the devil's assistant. The idea that witchcraft could be used to make other people mad was current in court circles in the late fourteenth and early fifteenth centuries, when the French nobility was seeking an explanation for Charles VI's madness.[170] Indeed, when Jean sans Peur, duke of Burgundy, arranged for the murder of Louis, duke of Orléans and brother of the king, he justified the act by accusing Louis of causing Charles VI's madness with the aid of sorcerers.[171] Many scholars have addressed the burgeoning interest in sorcery in the mid-fifteenth century, suggesting that popular belief and elite concern were coming together at this time.[172] The belief that sorcery could cause illness and particularly madness was developed further in fifteenth-century treatises by Johannes Nider and Heinrich Institoris.[173] It is possible that the supplicants seeking remission were aware of these shifting attitudes in religious and intellectual circles from sermons, and certainly the royal notaries would have been familiar with the treatises and their impact on legal discourse.

Bewitchment by a sorcerer was mentioned as a source of madness increasingly from the middle of the fifteenth century.[174] The earliest reference to sorcery in a letter about madness appeared in 1404, when a man suffering from the falling sickness (*caduc*) that caused him to become 'furieux et fol' chased a woman and beat her to death with a rock, screaming, 'old whore, you have bewitched [*encaraté*] me'.[175] However, it was not until the 1450s that sorcerers appeared in the remission letters as directly causing madness.[176] These later letters blamed sorcerers for having caused mad or possessed behavior and were generally not written on behalf of the mad person, who usually had not committed any crime, but rather for the mad person's family and neighbors who had sought out a renowned sorcerer and killed him or her

170 Bellaguet 1842, vol. 2, pp. 24–25.

171 Coville 1932 published an excerpt from Jean Petit's *Justification* on pages 314–315. See also Veenstra 1998, pp. 36–67 for a discussion of Petit's work in the context of the Dukes of Burgundy and their interest in sorcery.

172 See the articles in Jolly, Raudvere, and Peters 2002; Paravy 1979; and of course the seminal studies from the 1970s, Russell 1972 and Cohn 1975.

173 Institoris and Sprenger 2006; Nider 1999. These texts and the killing of witches are discussed in more detail in Pfau 2013a.

174 For more on this topic, see my essay, Pfau 2013a, pp. 50–71. This fits the chronology of witchcraft literature. See especially Cohn 1975; Jolly, Raudvere, and Peters 2002; Russell 1972.

175 AN JJ 158 fo 168 no 360, edited in Guérin 1909, vol. 8, pp. 38–41: 'furious and mad'; 'Pute veille, tu m'as encaraté'.

176 See AN JJ 181 fo 67v no 123 (in 1452); AN JJ 182 fo 51 no 85 (in 1453); AN JJ 182 fo 53 no 88 (in 1453); and AN JJ 182 fo 53v no 90 (in 1453) for the earliest cases I found.

in an attempt to break the spell. Sorcery led one girl in 1457 to 'run crazily [*folle*] around the fields completely naked'[177] and a man in 1480 to become 'hors du sens et memoire' and impotent.[178] The language used to describe madness caused by a sorcerer did not differ in any way from the language used to describe madness that developed from other causes.

The religious, literary, and political spheres in which the notaries interacted with each other and with other intellectuals may not have had a direct impact on their work in the royal chancery, but they were able to bring to bear their own knowledge of the significance of madness and possession in the political arena. There were times when determining whether a person suffered from a natural illness or a supernatural possession was absolutely central to the work undertaken, but there were also times when vocabulary could be flexible, and such considerations were insignificant.

In their attempts to find a conceptual vocabulary about madness, the composers of remission letters had a number of different cultural resources from which to draw. The language used to describe madness in remission letters varied widely, using multiple discourses in many different constellations and creating a fluid vision of the nature of madness. Most of the supplicants for remission described themselves as poor manual laborers and were most likely illiterate. The royal notaries, in contrast, were not only literate, but active in literary circles and a few were members of the French humanist movement.[179] It was thus in the interstices of discourse that the remission letters were composed. The language used is often vague and repetitious, but these iterations signal different contexts for understanding madness.

The notaries and supplicants who composed remission letters engaged in the process of constructing their concepts of madness through language.[180] The fluidity of possible terminology and definitions allowed for different levels of madness to emerge within and between remission letters. This spectrum of madness ranged from foolishness or stupidity all the way to insanity or murderous rage. Remission letters used a number of terms to

177 AN JJ 187 fo 89v no 173: 'courroit folle parmy les champs toute nue'.

178 AN JJ 208 fo 11 no 20: 'out of his senses and memory'.

179 Famiglietti 2004, p. 34.

180 There has been an increasing interest in the ways notaries in this period were shaping how people defined things, through the writing of wills, contracts, and other legal documents like remission letters. As Daniel Smail notes, 'by the mid-fourteenth century few people, certainly few propertied people, went through life without encountering the notaries in some official capacity on one or more occasions. [...] Despite this contact, notaries are not credited, as are the clergy, with a role in the shaping of western European culture and society'. Smail 2000, p. 23.

discuss madness. Because madness is a contested state that is so often defined in oppositional terms, it opens up discursive possibilities by forcing writers to consider the human capacity for reason, the danger of the melancholic temperament, or the mental and physical capabilities necessary to interact with others in acceptable ways.

In seeking a vocabulary to describe Jehannecte Troppé's troubling behavior, Jean de Rinel and the Troppé family were able to draw not only from the language of insanity that would have been familiar to Jehannecte's neighbors. Jean de Rinel, as part of a larger network of notaries who were active consumers of the French translations of Latin works, was able to use French terms that accessed a learned tradition. Though he and his fellow notaries may have been constrained by the legal framework of these remission letters, they were still influenced by their learned communities in the terms they chose to deploy and the kinds of knowledge those terms allowed them to claim. The next chapter focuses on the stories they chose to tell, and particularly the disruptions caused by people identified as mad.

2. Madness as Communal Threat

Abstract

The narrative structures used in remission letters demonstrate how the family advocated for the mad person by constructing stories about the crime, but also reveal details about the person's entire life. The evidence provided for mental illness earlier in the person's life was often idiosyncratic, and sometimes the narratives tried to provide logical linkages between the earlier behavior and the ultimate crime of the mad person. These individual narratives reveal a wide spectrum of beliefs about what caused madness and what kinds of behaviors and criminal acts were coded as mad. Although each narrative was distinct, a clear pattern emerges whereby the actions of the individual identified as mad disrupt familial and communal bonds.

Keyterms: Narrative, Crime, Insanity Defense, Community

In October of 1380, one month after Jehan de Moustier murdered his father, his 'close family'[1] sought a letter of remission for him. Jehan was in prison in the town of Saint Denis, from which the family traveled the short distance of twelve and a half kilometers to the royal capital, where Louis of Anjou was serving as regent for the eleven-year-old Charles VI. With the help of the notary P. de Disery, the family composed a letter explaining Jehan's crime and asking that he be pardoned. While in Jehannecte Troppé's narrative it is not clear whether her family had already decided to characterize her actions in terms of madness before meeting with the royal notary, in this particular case the family had already publicly identified Jehan de Moustier as mad. The remission letter explains that Jehan's condition had been recognized as madness by the local authorities, referring to a previous intervention by the Marshall of Pontoise, who provided the family with

1 AN JJ 118 fo 18v no 18: 'amis charnelx'. For a discussion of the meaning of 'parens et amis charnels', see Gauvard 1991, vol. 1, pp. 643–651.

Pfau, A., *Medieval Communities and the Mad: Narratives of Crime and Mental Illness in Late Medieval France*. Taylor & Francis Group, 2021
DOI: 10.5117/9789462983359_CH02

chains to help them control Jehan.[2] In the letter the supplicants and the notary considered the events of his life to highlight evidence of madness and construct a convincing narrative of his patricide that would then be read out in the local courts. Such a narrative had to be sufficiently compelling to be accepted and confirmed by both the king's council and the adverse party, who was given the opportunity to challenge the letter when it was read aloud by the local judge.[3]

Most remission letters sought to construct a coherent narrative of a particular crime. Letters composed on behalf of the mad, in contrast, generally sought to establish that the individual was indeed mad, and thus provided a narrative of a life. These biographies in miniature either involved evidence of an ongoing struggle with madness over the course of the individual's life or attempted to demonstrate the way madness caused the person to behave in unexpected ways, rupturing a recognizable identity that was constructed in part through kin and communal ties. This chapter explores the narrative structures of these letters, looking particularly at the ways in which the composers of these letters saw the crimes committed by the mad as particularly threatening to kin and community.

It is important to remember that letters of remission were joint efforts, co-authored by the supplicants and the royal notaries who recorded them. It is possible to speculate on what content was contributed by which 'composer'.[4] Clearly the royal notary who recorded the letters in the chancery archive was responsible for the formulaic language invoking the king's grace and mercy. The narrative of the crime and the life of the accused were at least in part supplied by the supplicants, who may have been responding to appropriate questions posed by the notary. While some letters for mad people who had recovered their sanity follow the more general pattern of remission letters sought by the individual who committed the crime, the majority was sought through the cooperative effort of the family as the mad person languished in prison awaiting trial or was detained due to the disease. The supplicants may even have consulted with a legal expert before coming to Paris in order to establish whether the case was eligible for remission. Once a letter of remission was received it had to be read aloud in the presence of the adverse party. Since the other side was granted the

2 AN JJ 118 fo 18v no 18.

3 Texier 1984, p. 9, p. 263 and pp. 324–338. Texier notes that this right to challenge did not negate royal authority. Although the victim could appeal the remission letter, it had to be done in front of a royal judge, thereby reaffirming royal judiciary power.

4 Davis 1987, pp. 15–19; Gauvard 1991, vol. 1, p. 66.

opportunity to dispute the narrative contained in the letter, it is conceivable that they also were involved in the composition. The supplicants may have come to an agreement with their adversaries before deciding to invest time and money in a trip to Paris to seek the king's pardon. Thus, many different minds were involved in defining and indicating madness within these letters.

This group, made up of legally-trained notaries, legal experts, supplicants seeking remission, and in some cases the adverse party, can be imagined in terms of a 'textual community', formed around a text, where one or more literate individuals provided access to that text for the larger, illiterate component.[5] The literate and knowledgeable experts provided a framework within which the information supplied by the supplicants could be given shape and meaning. As noted in the introduction, the invocation of madness was not common, but it does appear rarely but consistently over the one hundred fifty year period under examination.[6] Unlike the more common crimes, it seems that notaries did not develop a standard form for writing about crimes committed by the mad. Nevertheless, the notaries' knowledge about law codes gave them an awareness of the benefits and the hazards of establishing that a person was mad when he or she committed a crime,[7] as well as a general concept of what kind of evidence was necessary to demonstrate madness. Together with the supplicants, the notaries were able to construct a narrative that reflected on the life of the individual, providing convincing evidence of madness and building to the moment of the criminal act.

These narratives provide only one side of the story, although it is possible that the adverse party agreed to the pardon beforehand and thus had some control over the content of the letter. Nevertheless, remission letters conceal multiple alternative narratives that cannot be recovered, at the same time as they reveal a complex and compelling story. Bearing in mind that these

5 Brian Stock coined this term as a way of describing heretical communities in Europe, that centered around an interpreter who read aloud from texts. I have altered his use of the term: whereas the textual communities he describes were centered around pre-existing texts, the textual communities I am imagining are centered around the creation of a new text. See Stock 1990, p. 13.

6 On average, letters about madness appear in one percent of the total remission letters, and in the books that were fully examined they never exceeded three percent. On the other hand, only two of the thirty-five books searched yielded no references to madness.

7 Roman law established that mad people should not be held responsible for committing crimes. However, a number of French customals called for the mad to be restrained so as to prevent them from committing crimes. Some remission letters reflect these laws. See, for example, AN JJ 118 fo 18v no 18 (in 1380) and AN JJ 173 fo 33v no 63 (in 1425), edited in Le Cacheux 1907–1908, pp. 181–183.

letters were carefully constructed by a group of composers, and the resulting narrative had to be acceptable to all parties involved, how was Jehan de Moustier's particular narrative constructed? What mechanisms did his close family and the notary use to establish his madness and demonstrate that he could not be held responsible for the death of his father? What types of crimes were associated with madness and what can that tell us about how madness was understood?

I. Reconstructing a Life Narrative

Jehan de Moustier's letter of remission states that during the month of May 1379, he began to exhibit behaviors that his family interpreted as madness. The composers of his letter claimed that he 'was utterly mad as is apparent by his crimes'.[8] First, he 'took himself to the woods and the fields, whistling to the birds and running. He remained there for two or three days such that he should perish from hunger, and the good people who found him brought him back'.[9] After Jehan had repeated this behavior a few times, his father, Perrim, decided to take him to the shrine of Saint Titenerd at Gournay, north of Saint-Denis.[10] At the saint's shrine, he was chained up and left to await God's mercy. Escaping from those chains, he was recaptured and held with two sets of chains, but he escaped from those as well, demonstrating an abnormal strength.

When Jehan returned from the shrine, he was better for a time, but at the beginning of Lent in 1380 he began again to exhibit mad behavior, and the Marshal of Pontoise provided a particularly heavy set of chains to his father so that he could be controlled.[11] When he broke out of that set, 'a thing that did not seem possible for a man to do', his father refused to rechain him.[12] Once freed, Jehan proceeded to kill a heifer during the first week of Lent, which his family referenced as further proof of his madness. His final and

8 AN JJ 118 fo 18v no 18: 'soit pur fol comme il est apparu par ses crimes'.

9 AN JJ 118 fo 18v no 18: 'sen aloit par bois et par champs sifflant aus oiseaux coursent en demourant deux ou trois jours tant que il perissoix de faim et le ramenoient les bonnes genz qui le trouvoient'.

10 Neither I nor anyone with whom I have discussed this letter have ever heard of a Saint Titenerd. Indeed, the parish church in Gournay-sur-Marne is dedicated to Saint Arnoult.

11 In this case, the *mareschal* was most likely 'an officer of a court of law responsible for the custody of prisoners and for the keeping of order, and frequently entrusted with the keeping of a prison' as defined by the Oxford English Dictionary, which cites the earliest reference around 1300.

12 AN JJ 118 fo 18v no 18: 'qui ne sembloit pas possible chose afaire a homme'.

most serious crime also centered on food production: during a particularly hot week in September of the same year, the town mandated that anyone wanting to make bread needed to allow it to rise on Wednesday night and knead it on Thursday. However, Jehan decided to begin making the bread at nones (around 3 p.m.) instead of waiting until the late evening, because he wanted to knead the bread that night, not the next day. Perrim prevented him from doing so on Wednesday, but the next morning asked him if he was going to knead the bread. Jehan, in a fit of rage brought on, according to the composers of his letter, partly by his madness and partly by anger that he had not been allowed to knead the bread the night before, picked up 'a stick called a "basuche" with which one trims the vines'[13] and hit his father with it until he died. When the local justice arrived and told him 'you have killed your father', Jehan responded 'he was only my father according to whispers'.[14] The composers of Jehan's letter explained that they did not merely fear for his life, but also for his immortal soul, since 'if he were to suffer death for this, he does not have the memory or sense to recognize his creator'.[15]

The composers of this letter did not specify a primary cause of Jehan de Moustier's madness, but it is clear they made connections between the events they noticed as unusual and the ultimate crime he committed. In beginning to describe his madness, the letter composers emphasized that it was apparent from his 'crimes'. Although his final 'crime' was the murder of his father, his earlier acts appear less serious than that, particularly to a modern eye, but the composers of Jehan's remission letter viewed these other events as 'crimes' as well. In this letter, criminal acts were caused by madness, and simultaneously provided proof that the criminal was mad, creating a circular logic that went uncontested. While there is an intimate connection between crime and madness in these remission letters, there was no single definition of what constituted a mad crime, which makes these texts so interesting. In Jehan de Moustier's case, his mad behavior followed a particular and distinct pattern that centered on food production and consumption.

13 AN JJ 118 fo 18v no 18: 'un baston appelle basuche dont on prongue les vignes'.

14 AN JJ 118 fo 18v no 18: 'tu as tue ton pere il dist que il nestoit son pere que dans oreille'. I have chosen to translate 'dans oreille' here as 'according to whispers' because it resonates better than 'in the ear'. I have not been able to find proof that this is, in fact, a good colloquial translation, despite searching for a similar usage elsewhere, so I have chosen not to fully pursue this particular episode in Jehan de Moustier's letter, although the inability to recognize familial relationships does seem to be an important facet of medieval conceptions of madness.

15 AN JJ 118 fo 18v no 18: 'se pour ce il souffroit mort il navroit memoire ne senz de recognoistre son createur'.

From Jehan's letter it is possible to extract a compelling narrative of escalating mad behavior. Jehan's first episode of madness involved an inability to care for himself, as he ran through the fields and woods and did not eat anything for several days. The trope of the mad person running in the fields would have been familiar from the biblical story of Nebuchadnezzar and literary figures such as the Arthurian heroes Yvain and Lancelot. Running in the fields was in fact used as a proof of madness in some other remission letters,[16] but the mention of a lack of sustenance was unusual. Where the biblical figure Nebuchadnezzar ate grass[17] and Chrétien de Troyes' Arthurian knight Yvain ate raw meat,[18] Jehan de Moustier engaged in 'unholy anorexia'.[19] Indeed, when he was finally captured and returned to the village, his family asserted that he was nearly dead from hunger. Jehan's starvation to the point of death strongly suggested that his inability to feed and care for himself threatened his own life.

This reference to Jehan's excessive starvation is particularly interesting in light of Jean Gerson's contemporary attempts to limit what he saw as the excessive fasting that many female mystics were practicing, as discussed above.[20] As he explained, the dangers of excessive fasting are physiological. Starvation can cause mania, rage, or melancholy to such an extent that visions occur, and create a false image of reality. Gerson's theory connecting food consumption to madness may have been influenced by a wider social

16 For example, a sorcerer made people run through the fields because of madness in AN JJ 187 fo 89v no 173 (in 1457) and AN JJ 208 fo 11 no 20 (in 1480). A young boy who was guilty of theft was similarly known to run through the fields due to his madness in AN JJ 196 fo 192 no 307 (in 1470), as was a man who later committed murder in AN JJ 229 fo 22v no 44 (in 1497).

17 Daniel 4:30.

18 The consumption of uncooked food is held up as a proof of madness in Chretien de Troyes' tale. See Chrétien de Troyes 1994, p. 274.

19 Here I am playing on Rudolph Bell's concept of 'holy anorexia' in Bell 1985. His work is controversial, and Carolyn Walker Bynum has done much to challenge his perspective, arguing that control of food was a way in which women empowered themselves. See Bynum 1987. It is also necessary to note the more recent contribution to this debate by Nancy Caciola 2003. Caciola argues that Bynum and others have overemphasized the hagiographical views of the confessors who wrote these women's lives. She contends that any examination of these women's actions has to take into account the fact that they were seldom sanctioned by the church, and that the larger population viewed them with serious suspicion. However, Caciola focuses solely on Gerson's distinction between divine and demonic inspiration. While this was admittedly Gerson's main focus, his acknowledgement of mental disturbance is also significant.

20 Gerson 1998, pp. 334–364. Although there is no direct evidence that royal notaries were interested in Gerson's theological works, some of them were involved in epistolary communication with him in the debate over the *Roman de la Rose*, and may have been aware of his other projects. Certainly the notaries, as educated men living in Paris, can be credited with an awareness of the larger discourse around discernment in this period.

belief. The composers of Jehan de Moustier's letter seemed to believe that his madness caused him to starve himself, thereby exacerbating his madness and forming the same dangerous cycle.

In a second episode, after a period of sanity, Jehan de Moustier killed a heifer during Lent. This was doubly problematic, and simultaneously violated both implicit and explicit rules governing animal slaughter in a medieval village. A heifer is a cow that has not yet calved and Lent was a time when no one was supposed to eat it, so the slaughtered cow would be wasted. A cow, but especially a cow that could be expected to produce other cows, was a valuable commodity for a household. There is evidence from the records of medieval estates, as well as archaeological evidence from the waste deposits of both estates and cities, suggesting that young, female animals that had not yet reproduced were not slaughtered, even by the wealthy.[21] Similarly, although the major period for slaughter, especially of pigs but also of cows, was in late fall and early winter, animals were generally killed and taken to market in towns and cities throughout the year, except during Lent.[22] The slaughter of this particular animal at this particular time, according to the composers of the letter, provided proof of the return of Jehan de Moustier's madness, which in this case was characterized as prodigality. His wasteful behavior threatened his family's food store, since he killed the cow before it had produced a new generation and when it could not be consumed.

In the final episode recorded in the letter, he killed his father over a dispute about when to knead bread. In this case, Jehan de Moustier's desire to knead the bread early was a threat to the community as a whole. The heat of the summer had caused fevers and illness in the town, and the decision to bake bread in the communal oven on a certain day and at a certain time was intended to protect the community from the excessive heat of baking.[23] Jehan's

21 Kathleen Biddick 1989 used records from Peterborough Abbey in England and found, as might be expected, that female cows were not slaughtered until after they had reproduced, although males might be slaughtered young. See also Doll 2003, p. 283. Doll looked at digs from towns, castles, monasteries, and sewers in Germany from the thirteenth to the seventeenth centuries, and found that seventy to ninety percent of slaughtered animals were two years old or more.

22 In a study of butchery records in two Italian towns, Gillian Clarke found that no animal's meat was sold during Lent. Clarke 1992, especially the tables on pp. 78–79. December was the month of slaughter in medieval calendars, and the butchers' records studied by Clarke suggest there was an increase in late fall and early winter, but there does not seem to be a single month for slaughter. For the calendars, see Henisch 1999, p. 127. Interestingly, she sees a shift in the late fifteenth century towards images of buying meat in town, instead of images of slaughtering, but nevertheless the image of the animal 'harvest' is generally in December.

23 For more on communal ovens, see Bloch 1967, p. 153.

attempt to knead the bread early would have ruined the family's bread, but the further implications of his desire to bake the bread at an inappropriate time would have been even more serious in the eyes of his neighbors. Clearly, Jehan's inability to comprehend both the simple and the complex relationships to food that were apparent to everyone else in his village led to serious problems, for his own health and that of others. The narrative of food production and consumption builds as the 'crimes' build, to a climax where Jehan de Moustier threatened the community's welfare and ultimately killed his father.

In attempting to comprehend a crime that appears inexplicable, the composers of remission letters for the mad reinterpreted the past of the individual, seeking a point of rupture where the person moved from sanity to madness. This approach is similar to that used in hagiographical writings, where the saint's later sanctity is allowed to bleed back into their childhood.[24] It is clear in the letter for Jehan de Moustier that madness was inscribed through a certain pattern of behaviors that was recalled as constituting a rupture between expected and actual acts. The retrospective consideration of Jehan's actions in terms of his final crime allowed the composers of his remission letter to find a rationale for his behavior. The ways in which madness is described and determined is embedded within the rhythm of medieval village culture, where food production and consumption were central to everyday life. The composers of Jehan de Moustier's remission letter did not concern themselves with medical or psychological causes of madness; rather their description of his inexplicable behavior sought a source for madness in terms of social interactions. By 'making sense' of the 'insensible' through the development of a clear pattern only visible in retrospect, the composers created a narrative whereby Jehan's final crime was comprehensible. In turning now to the larger corpus of letters, this chapter will consider how the crimes committed by the mad were understood as particularly damaging to the community.

II. Moments of Rupture: Crimes Against the Family and the Community

As discussed in Chapter One, remission letters mediated between popular beliefs about madness held by the family telling the story and elite knowledge held by the notary writing the letter. In a process of cooperative composition,

24 Many of the saints in Jacobus de Voragine's *Golden Legend*, for example, are described as having exemplarily holy childhoods. Jacobus de Voragine 1993.

the letter was written both for the king's council, who had to ratify it, and for the adverse party, who had to approve its content in front of the judge.[25] Thus, the information contained had to be comprehensible on many levels. Family members advocated for the mad by attempting to understand and explain madness, both as it existed inside the body and as it was externally performed.[26] In an effort to describe behavior they perceived as a sign of madness, the composers of remission letters wrote life histories of the mad, explaining actions in light of or in extreme contrast to the actions of madness.

Madness is often seen as the rupture of an identity, constructed through kin and communal ties, that can be perceived through certain actions signaling a shift between the person's sane behavior and mad behavior. Sylvia Huot, in discussing madness in medieval French literature, argues that

> [s]anity is the perfect concordance of a symbolically constituted identity, the performance through which that identity is staged, and the body that gives it material form; and madness can be understood as the dissolution of that construct. The onset of madness results in an incoherent relationship between body, performance, and social identity.[27]

These 'incoherent relationships' are defined and explored in remission letters as they are in the literary texts Huot references. The causes of madness and the resultant behavior of the mad were both interpreted in terms that the family members composing the letter could access, and these terms described an individual who acted in a way that was no longer recognizable as part of the social identity the mad person had previously enacted. Madness was an observable phenomenon, defined through social interactions and perceptions. As is clear from Jehan de Moustier's letter, which revolved around food consumption and production, the specific patterns of individual cases were focused within their particular narrative. The letters all represented the individual's madness as a danger to the surrounding community, occasionally just at the moment of the crime, but often for an extended period beforehand.

25 Gauvard 1991, vol. 1, p. 67.

26 In talking about the performance of madness I am not trying to suggest these people were falsely claiming to be insane, but rather highlighting the fact that the interiority of madness as a disease can never be accessed, leaving only the external signs of madness as an indicator of the internal state. Thus, madness is performed and interpreted. See Caciola 2000, pp. 287–290 for a discussion of these ideas as they relate to spirit possession.

27 Huot 2003, p. 182.

Although there was no single required pattern for telling a narrative of mad crime, certain types of information were included in most of these letters. The kinds of narrative arcs used in the letters inscribed a number of shared beliefs about madness. Remission letters about the mad reflected the same kinds of conflicting images of madness that appeared in the legal discourse of the time. Mad people were simultaneously feared for the threat they represented (and most often, in the letters, had already carried out) and considered in need of protection from the repercussions of their actions.[28] The most common fear that remission letters revealed was that mad people would attack family members or themselves. The crimes of the mad were focused inside the household, rather than outside, which distinguished them from the usual crimes for which remission was sought. This may reflect a cultural perception of intrafamilial crime as more serious than interfamilial crime. Indeed, one of the few crimes that were theoretically considered 'irremissible' was parricide, showing continuity with the Roman perspective that saw the murder of a family member as particularly troublesome.[29] Not all remission letters for parricide referred to madness as a mitigating factor,[30] but there is a suggestive pattern to the types of crime viewed as outside the realm of reason.

Every letter of remission began with the implicit acknowledgement that a crime had been committed, but the revelation of the crime was delayed until the culmination of the narration. That said, some letters foreshadowed the nature of the crime through particular phrases. For example, often

28 Philippe de Beaumanoir, for example, maintained: 'Those who are insane [*forsené*] should be bound by those who must guard them and everyone must help do this to avoid the damages that might come from them, for they could quickly kill themselves and others'. Philippe de Beaumanoir 1970–1974, vol. 2, ch. 52, paragraph 1575: 'Cil qui sont forsené doivent estre lié par ceus qui les doivent garder et chascuns doit aidier a ce fere pour eschiver les damages qui par aus pueent venir, car tost ociroient aus et autrui'.

29 Mommsen, Krueger, and Watson 1985, vol. 4, p. 822, book 48.9: 'Truly, if anyone kills a parent in a fit of madness, he shall not be punished, as the deified brothers wrote in a rescript in the case of a man who had killed his mother in a fit of madness; for it was enough for him to be punished by the madness itself.' 'Sane si per furorem aliquis parentem occiderit, inpunitus erit, ut diui fratres rescripserunt super eo, qui per furorem matrem necauerat: nam sufficere furore ipso eum puniri.' Esther Cohen argues, on the basis of rhetoric about remission letters in royal charters rather than on the basis of the content of remission letters themselves, that 'genuinely heinous crimes (such as parricide) neither deserved nor received pardon'. Cohen 1993, p. 50. Clearly, the ideal did not match up to the real regarding parricide.

30 See the tables in Gauvard 1991, vol. 2, pp. 614–620.

an individual was introduced as 'the late'[31] so-and-so, generally (although not always) indicating that that person would lose his or her life in the course of the narrated events. Indeed, often a clear indication of suicide was the linkage of 'the late' with the name of the individual on behalf of whom the remission was being sought. The particular types of crimes committed by mad perpetrators signaled a departure from expected behavior, though sometimes details recalled from the past that established the onset and development of the perpetrator's madness foreshadowed the ultimate crime, as the letter for Jehan de Moustier demonstrates. All remission narratives were constructed around the moment of a crime. Although the accused perpetrator did not admit his or her guilt in every case, nevertheless a description of the crime of which the supplicant was accused appeared in every letter. Every type of crime committed by a person labeled as mad in remission letters also appeared in other letters committed by a sane person. However, there are patterns to the crimes associated with madness that go beyond the surface of the act committed. These were acts that were particularly damaging to the family or the community of the mad person. The association of madness with crimes targeting people or things that should be protected has also been shown by Michael MacDonald in his study of seventeenth-century England.[32] These crimes were not described as random, but rather as disruptive of important social and familial ties.

Perceptions of madness both affected and were affected by the particular crimes associated with mad criminals. No crimes were considered exclusively 'mad crimes'.[33] However, while the basic crime is the same, the details in the letters reveal particular ways in which crimes committed by the mad were distinctive. The majority of these crimes acted against the mad person's own identity or against his or her family.[34] These types of crimes were troubling to the family and the royal notary who worked together to compose these letters, and this discomfort translated itself into the description of the mad person and the crime committed.

31 *Feu* or *feue*.

32 MacDonald 1981.

33 Indeed, it is worth pointing out that many of these crimes were those Gauvard refers to as 'stereotypes of serious crimes'. See Gauvard 1999, pp. 1–48.

34 Identity is being constructed through these letters in terms of the individuals' relationship to others, particularly their participation in groups, specifically family and community. I am basing this partly on Caroline Walker Bynum's description of identity construction in the twelfth century, Bynum 1984. See also Heers 1977, pp. 1–15.

Table 2 Crimes of the mad

Crime	Number	Percentage of Total	Male	Female
Arson	9	5.8%	5	4
Bestiality	3	2%	3	0
Blasphemy[35]	5	3.2%	5	0
Cause of Murder	8	5.2%	1	7
Infanticide	7	4.5%	1	6
Murder	35	22.5%	29	6
Rape[36]	3	2%	3	0
Suicide	18	11.6%	8	10
Theft	27	17.4%	19	8
Treason	11	7%	11	0
Victim of Crime	20	13%	13	7
Other	9	5.8%	6	3
Total	155		104	51

Murders of Family and Neighbors

The crime of murder was disruptive to a community, regardless of the mental state of the perpetrator. Murder had the potential to spiral into a feud with an extended kin network and sometimes the entire neighborhood taking sides.[37] Remission letters, read out loud in front of the adverse party and open to objection, could play a role of mediation between the two sides, clarifying the case from the perspective of the criminal and attempting to temper the anger of the surviving family. Indeed, murder was the most common crime for which to seek remission in general. Claude Gauvard, in her study of remission letters, argues that when an attempt was made in 1400 to curb the number of remissions being granted, the letters became more focused on homicide as the particular crime for which remission

35 Charles VI passed a number of laws against blasphemy during his reign. The first was recorded in Parlement in 1397. Stein 1908, 153–154. When he reconfirmed the law in 1415, the mad king included language suggesting that the problems of the realm might have their roots in the blasphemy of the people, saying 'it may be for this cause that many great disgraces and inconveniences have come and come every day in diverse ways, to Us and to our said subjects' ('puet estre que à ceste cause pluseurs grans esclandres & inconveniens qui sont avenuz & aviennent de jour en jour en diverses manieres, sur Nous & nosdiz subgiez'). Vilevault and Bréquigny 1763, 243.

36 There are very few rape cases that mention madness, though there are considerably more rape cases in letters of remission as a whole. For more, see Gauvard 1991, vol. 1, 330–339; Prevenier 1990; and Prevenier 1999.

37 See for example, Meyerson 2004; Muchembled 1989; and Muir 1993.

should be granted.[38] Whereas my own numerical study of remission letters suggests that Gauvard is mistaken in her assessment of the impact of this regulation,[39] homicides certainly did account for a large percentage of the letters from the time when they were first instituted, and the percentage increased over time. Of the 155 letters about mad people examined for this study, thirty-five provided remission for murder, making up the highest percentage.[40] The narratives of murder cases involving mad people were different from the more common passionate, drunken murders, however. In most cases, mad people murdered friends or family members. While these types of murders could be committed by sane people, the pattern is still suggestive of a larger concept of the relationship between madness and crime. Roman law established that mad people should not be held responsible for parricide, creating a direct link between madness and intrafamilial murder.[41] Indeed, in these remission letters mad people seldom appeared lashing out at complete strangers, and when they did it was usually in the context of the stranger seeking remission for having killed the mad person, rather than the other way around.[42] The murder of close companions and family members was seen as a particularly disturbing act, and, in cases where there were other recognizable factors that contributed (if only in retrospect) to the medieval image of madness, such a murderer could be viewed as mentally disturbed.[43]

In eighteen of the cases of murder by a mad person, the victim was a member of the murderer's family. Most of these involved the murder of a spouse, although there were also several cases of murder across generations, where the victim was the father, mother-in-law (but never the

38 Gauvard 1991, vol. 1, p. 64.

39 Gauvard 1991 uses the numerical decrease to make her argument, but remission letters remain as the same percentage of total chancery business, suggesting it is not a decrease in the granting of remission that is being marked but a decrease in the use of the chancery. Given that this decrease occurs during a period of civil war and governmental instability due to Charles VI's madness, it seems more likely that this general upheaval, rather than a targeted effort to limit remissable crimes, caused the numerical decrease in remissions granted.

40 Wendy Turner also found that homicide 'was the most commonly prosecuted crime involving the mentally incapacitated' in England. Turner 2013a, p. 114.

41 Mommsen, Krueger, and Watson 1985, vol. 4, p. 822, Book 48.9

42 For example, AN JJ 89 fo 142v no 340 (in 1357); AN JJ 172 fo 113v no 221 (in 1422); and AN JJ 219 fo 132 no 216 (in 1488).

43 Both Claude Gauvard and Barbara Hanawalt have looked at murders between relatives in France and England, respectively. See Gauvard 1991, vol. 2, p. 573 for her discussion of violence between married couples, which she found to compose only 2% of cases. Hanawalt notes that '[a]bout a third of the intra-familial homicide cases tried in gaol delivery were committed by the insane'. Hanawalt 1974, p. 11.

mother), father-in-law, or uncle.[44] These murders most often occurred in the household, combining both relationships and spaces where murder was jarringly unexpected. Unlike the public tavern, where drunken arguments could lead to accidental murder with the daggers and knives carried by most people,[45] murders in the household were seen as disruptive. Even the weapons chosen carried added significance. Household murderers picked up whatever weapon happened to be lying around, often an axe used to chop wood or a stick with iron on the end of it, such as a utensil used to trim vines or a hoe. The letters always specified the quotidian use of these household items, clearly indicating that the crime was not premeditated and that the murder weapon was easily at hand, and not a weapon, such as a sword, intended for use only in violence approved by the king.[46]

Several of the murder cases took place in the middle of the night, a common time for murder according to other studies of medieval crime.[47] However, these murders did not follow the usual pattern of nighttime homicides that took place outside. Rather, most took place in the household, and often between people sleeping in the same bed. In 1392, for example, Pierre le Bagnaudel, who 'was often furious, lunatic and out of his memory',[48] went to bed one Sunday night, and woke up again in the early hours of Monday morning in a state of madness. He beat his wife with a hoe, then got back into bed beside her and slept until morning, still holding the murder weapon. Pierre le Bagnaudel's lack of recognition of his actions and the fact that he remained beside the mortally wounded body of his wife, holding the murder weapon in his hand, rather than running away, were pointed out by his family as further indications of madness.[49] A similar story from 1425, discussed above, described the actions of Jehannecte Troppé, who woke up in the middle of the night seeing visions that led her to beat her husband. When she went back to bed, her husband woke her again and she was shocked when she lit a candle and saw his wounds. The letter specifies that she cared for her husband's wounds 'not knowing she had done the said

44 Those cases where the victim is the mad person's child will be treated separately, under infanticide, since such cases were categorized separately under medieval legal traditions.

45 Gonthier 1992, pp. 113–115.

46 The letters feel rather like a game of *Clue* as a result. 'It was Jehan de Moustier in the kitchen with the stick used to trim the vines'.

47 Nicole Gonthier notes that curfews were instated because night was seen as a time that 'peut cacher les criminels et favoriser leurs intentions perverses'. Gonthier 1998, pp. 53–55.

48 AN JJ 143 fo 108v no 207: 'souventeffoiz est fureur lunatiques et hors de son memoire'.

49 Voluntary exile after committing a crime was an accepted, and in some cases even expected, response.

deed'.[50] The marriage bed, unlike the public street, was a location in which violence was unexpected and disturbing, and this type of violent attack on a spouse who was sleeping ruptured the safe haven of the household.

Spouses were not the only possible victims of violence within the household. In 1376, the wife and family of Pierre de Solente explained that he was a seventy-year-old man who had suffered for about a year from the 'fragility or diminution of his body and of his sensuality' to such an extent that he had 'become entirely idiotic and also as if furious and out of his correct thoughts'.[51] Initially, his family was concerned that he would commit suicide by hanging or drowning himself, and his wife was careful to watch over him. However, one morning she left him sleeping with their nine-year-old son, Thomassin, so she could go to the market. Thomassin refused to get up when his father asked him to do so, arguing with his father and crying. In response, much like Jehan de Moustier, Pierre went significantly beyond what might be reasonable. In the letter, they explained he was 'moved by his madness, by evil temptation, seduced by the enemy of human creatures' such that he grabbed his son by the head and cut his throat with a knife.[52] Afterwards, Pierre tried again to drown himself but was stopped by his neighbors and his wife who had returned home. In contemplating his crime, the composers of his letter noted that he 'had forgotten the natural love that he must have for his said son'.[53] Pierre's murder of his son Thomassin clearly disrupted his community's expectations.

Even when the victim was not a member of the family, narratives that chose to deploy the language of madness were often about inexplicable and unexpected acts of violence that posed clear threats to the community. The story of Ysabeau, daughter of the Montpellier merchant Raymon Sarvallier, recorded in a letter from 1408, is a clear example of this. In many ways, Ysabeau's behavior ruptured social expectations, and it was this behavior that first caused her community to identify her as someone who 'does not have good, natural sense'.[54] During her first marriage to Naudin de Moscre, the son of the Sire de Moscre, Ysabeau only lived with her husband for a short time, and instead moved around her friends' homes without the

50 AN JJ 173 fo 33v no 63. Edited in Le Cacheux 1907–1908, vol. 1, pp. 181–183: 'non sachant avoir fait ledit fait'.

51 AN JJ 110 fo 125 no 108: 'fragilite ou diminucion de son corps et de sa sensualite soit devenu tout ydiote et aussi comme furieux hors de sa droit pensée'.

52 AN JJ 110 fo 125 no 108: 'meu en sa forcenerie par mauvaise temptacion seduit par lennemj dumaine creature'.

53 AN JJ 110 fo 125 no 108: 'avoit oblie lamour naturelle quil devoit avoir a son dit filz'.

54 AN JJ 163 fo 130 no 229: 'quelle navoit pas bon sens naturel'.

permission of her husband. After Naudin de Moscre's death, she married Guille Gauguin, and in the eleven years since her second marriage she had continued her peripatetic lifestyle, staying 'in the home of her mother and with her other friends by day and by night [...] without the permission and desire of her said husband'.[55] In some ways, then, Ysabeau's behavior followed the general pattern of a bad wife, though the composers of the letter written on her behalf were quick to assert that, even if she had been away from her husband overnight, she was an honest woman who had never been accused of adultery or fornication. Instead, as more proof of her disruptive behavior, they mentioned two occasions where she tried to drown herself in local wells, once at the convent of the Sisters of Saint Katherine. Fortunately, both times the 'good people' of Montpellier prevented her. As a result of these disruptive behaviors, Ysabeau 'was defamed in the said town of Montpellier and other places there where people knew of her' as a 'person who is not very sensible with good discretion or natural sense'.[56] So before she committed murder, Ysabeau was already recognized by her community as someone who might be a disruptive force. At this point, however, she had only damaged her marriages and threatened to harm herself.

In the end, Ysabeau's crime did not follow the pattern of her previous behavior, which made it unpredictable, so that her community could not have known she posed a danger to others. One day in April, she was in the solar of a house (not her husband's) when she called from the window to an eight-year-old servant girl who was passing by carrying bread and pastries for her master, Phot Ostarde. When the girl came to the window, Ysabeau picked up a pestle that was lying nearby and 'suddenly and as if insane and out of her good sense and natural discretion' hit the girl over the head.[57] As with several other cases where a mad person killed someone who was not a relative, the letter on behalf of Ysabeau clarified that she did not have any hatred for the girl or any of her connections nor had she engaged in any arguments with them. These assurances were used to locate this crime as an aberration, one that certainly did not spring from a premeditated revenge. As a result, the murder of the unnamed servant girl, who was just going about her business and trusted her neighbors, was all the more troubling because

55 AN JJ 163 fo 130 no 229: 'en lostel de sa mere et avec ses autres amis tant de jour comme de nuit et comme paravant sans congie et voulente de son dit mari'.

56 AN JJ 163 fo 130 no 229: 'elle est diffamer en la dit ville de Montpelier et autre part la ou len a congnoissance delle' 'comme personne qui nest pas bien sensible de bonne discrecion ou sens naturel'.

57 AN JJ 163 fo 130 no 229: 'incontinant et comme aliene et hors de son bon sens et discrecion naturelle'.

it was unexpected. Ysabeau's actions were unpredictable and endangered her community at large, not just her own life or her reputation.

In each of these cases of murder, the mad perpetrator violated expectations of safety that were in place due to kin relationships or neighborliness. Pierre le Bagnaudel's wife, Jehannecte Troppé's husband, and Pierre de Solente's son were all sleeping, trusting their family members would care for them. None of these relationships was described as unusually tense, except that the two Pierres and Jehannecte were known to have had episodes of madness previously. Similarly, Ysabeau Sarvallier's victim was going about her master's business, bringing home goods from the bakery, when she was called over to help a neighbor. Again, Ysabeau was known locally as a mad woman. However, much as Charles VI was allowed to govern the realm during his periods of sanity, Pierre, Jehannecte, Pierre, and Ysabeau were all allowed to continue in their usual roles despite the danger they ended up posing to others in their families or communities.

Theft in Inappropriate Circumstances

The second most common crime in letters for the mad was theft.[58] The invocation of madness tended to appear in letters where people had chosen inappropriate targets for their thefts, again disrupting expectations of safety, this time of goods. The narratives also described thefts that provided no material benefit for the perpetrator, who either threw away the stolen goods or had no knowledge of where they had hidden them. In these letters, the use of the rhetoric of madness was a more subtle indication of popular considerations of folly and, compared to murder cases, a less dangerous lack of sense.[59] However, some of these letters did represent the thief as threatening, shifting the terminology of madness from 'foolish' to 'furious', 'without good sense and understanding', and 'melancholy'.[60] In every case, the thefts described challenged communal expectations of who might steal from whom and why.

Many cases focused on the inadvisability of the particular theft committed. For example, a letter from 1428 described the actions of Marion Hodee, who stole from her master, the local captain of the guard. The relationship

58 This also follows the general pattern for remission letters as a whole. Theft made up 16% of total crimes in Gauvard's study. Gauvard 1991, vol. 1, p. 242, table 8.

59 See for example AN JJ 99 fo 173v no 567 (in 1368); AN JJ 106 fo 173 no 318 (in 1374); and AN JJ 106 fo 184v no 352 (in 1374).

60 See AN JJ 107 fo 193v no 377 (in 1375); AN JJ 115 fo 52 no 114 (in 1379); AN JJ 188 fo 82v no 163 (in 1459); and AN JJ 196 fo 192 no 307 (in 1470).

between the thief and her victim was a hierarchical one, and in addition his role as captain of the guard made him a dangerous target for any theft. As the letter composers explained, Marion had 'little understanding and was as if an idiot or insensible' and she acted 'without thinking she was doing wrong',[61] a characterization that in part sprang from her actions, which were clearly perceived as idiotic. The choice to steal from her employer was not well-considered, and it also raised fears that hierarchies might be challenged. In addition to the attempt to justify Marion's actions in terms of her lack of understanding, the letter explained that she was driven to steal from her master because her relative, Jehan Baptiste, wanted revenge on the captain for having dishonest relations with Jehan's wife. The complex social relationships involved in this narrative highlighted the difficulty of the situation for Marion. Her kinship with Jehan, a horizontal tie, led her to act against her master, with whom she had vertical ties. The whole situation arose because Marion's master had taken Jehan's wife as a mistress. Marion was exonerated, then, both because it was her kinsman's idea and because, being a simple and insensible woman, she did not know what she was doing was wrong. Indeed, as the letter explained, Marion was caught because she was witnessed throwing the goods she had stolen into the castle moat. The portrayal of Marion as mad held power because her crime could be recognized as ill-considered and lacking any personal benefit.

Many cases involving mad thieves present hierarchical relationships between the thief and his or her victim, suggesting these crimes were viewed as especially problematic. In a letter composed in 1387, Guillorz de la Cayroze humbly requested the release of his son, Perym. The young man, who was only fifteen at the time, had been arrested under suspicion of theft from a merchant staying in the inn that Guillorz de la Cayroze maintained in Angiers. The letter began as a straightforward tale about a merchant who left his well-filled purse in a sack in his room. During his absence, the purse was stolen, and he accused the innkeeper's son of theft. If Perym had been guilty, stealing from a guest at his father's inn would have violated expectations of safety. However, at this point, the letter's narrative became more complicated. Perym, after undergoing torture in prison, confessed he had taken the purse. First he claimed it was in the bed in the chamber where the merchants were staying, but when the authorities looked for it there, their search was fruitless. Perym then denied having taken the purse until they began to torture him again, at which point he again confessed,

61 AN JJ 174 fo 68v no 163: 'poy sachant et qui est comme ydiote ou insensee'; 'non cuidant mesprendre'.

providing them with a new hiding spot that again turned out to be empty. According to the letter, this wild goose chase continued for some time, and the money was never found. Guillorz used the remission letter to insist that his son should be released, 'considering the youth of the said Perym who is as if completely idiotic and does not have a good natural sense'.[62]

In Perym de la Cayroze's case, the composers of the remission letter constructed a complex narrative to explain why he should be released from prison. Unlike other letters that established the subject's madness from the beginning, here it was not raised until near the end of the letter. Instead, the letter began with a straightforward crime that only became troubling when the boy confessed. Through the structure of the narrative, it was Perym's many false confessions under torture that made his status as an idiot without good common sense believable. Aside from descriptions of Perym's own confessions, each of which was retracted after the torture was removed, nowhere does the letter admit Perym was guilty of stealing the money. In this way, the letter excused Perym on multiple levels. Other than his retracted confessions, there was no proof he had taken the money, and even if he had stolen it, his youth made such actions excusable, and his lack of sense made him immune to punishment.

Clearly sane thieves could and did also steal from their social superiors. However, as both of these cases indicate, the particularity of the relationships between thief and victim and therefore the potential damage to the thief's own livelihood or that of his or her kin due to the theft made these cases troubling. Both Marion Hodee's and Perym de la Cayroze's alleged victims had the power to pursue them. Both were suspects because they had access to the victims' belongings, but they also had much to lose by committing the theft. The crime itself could be construed as an act that violated Marion Hodee's and Perym de la Cayroze's positions in the community, as well as threatening their own or their family's livelihood. Perym's case simultaneously indicated the folly of the crime, which had already had an adverse effect on his father's business, and the foolishness of Perym, who confessed under torture to a crime that, his father insisted, he had not committed.

Homicide Against Themselves

Perhaps one of the most problematic targets of mad violence was the self. Indeed, as noted above, some of the letters about murder cited previous

62 AN JJ 130 fo 159 no 282: 'considerant aussi la jeuneses du dit pym qui est comme tout ydiot et na pas bon senz naturel'.

suicide attempts as proof of the person's madness. With eighteen of the 155 letters, suicide was the fourth most common crime for which families mentioned madness as an explanation, which shifts away from the pattern for remission letters in general.[63] Gauvard lists suicide as a mere 0.4% of the crimes committed in remission letters during Charles VI's reign,[64] whereas suicide makes up almost 12% of the crimes committed by mad people. Again, these letters highlighted problems of identity, family, and community.

In his study of suicide in the Middle Ages, Alexander Murray found that 'a suicide, or suicidal thought or act, follows an event of social dislocation, whether from crime, disgrace, or financial ruin'.[65] Many remission letters followed this pattern, describing a particular despair or an illness that brought on the decision to die. Suicide was considered both a religious sin and a civil crime in the Middle Ages. The Christian church, through the figure of Judas, informed people that suicides were damned for eternity. In medieval art, suicides were associated with the vice of Despair, usually paired with the virtue of Hope, first through the figure of Judas, and later with general suicidal figures, depicted either hanging from a rope like Judas or stabbing themselves with a knife.[66] Theologians took up this concept and further developed it. Augustine, for example, in *The City of God*, argued that suicide was a violation of the commandment 'thou shalt not kill'.[67] Thomas Aquinas, in his *Summa Theologica*, agreed that suicide was a sin. He expanded Augustine's evaluation of why, building on the idea that suicide violated this commandment, and arguing that suicide further violated natural love and charity, according to which man should love himself. Perhaps most significantly, Aquinas stated that 'every man is part of the community, so that he belongs to the community in virtue of what he is. Suicide therefore involves damaging the community'.[68] The concept that suicide injured the community as a whole by harming one member provides an interesting perspective on medieval laws against it. The secular government helped the church to regulate suicides by confiscating the body and the goods of suspected suicides. The body would not only be buried in unconsecrated ground, but would also be symbolically executed

63 The third most common reference to madness in remission letters was as a victim of crime, which will be discussed in more depth below.

64 Gauvard 1991, vol. 1, p. 242, table 8.

65 Murray 1998, vol. 1, p. 317.

66 See Barasch 1999 for an exploration of this phenomenon in art.

67 Augustine 1957, vol. 1, pp. 90–95, Book I.20.

68 Aquinas 1964, vol. 38, pp. 32–33, 2.2.64 Art. 5. 'homo est communitatis: et ita id quod est, est communitatis; unde in hoc quod seipsum interficit, injuriam communitati facit'.

by being hanged as a murderer. The suicide's goods were confiscated by the crown, often leaving the remaining family destitute as well as destroying their reputation and standing in the community.[69] As a result, suicide was a crime not only against the self and the community, but also against the surviving family.

Some remission letters focused solely on the dire situation of the innocent family members. In these letters, the suicide him- or herself played a small role, whereas the remaining family's size, economic needs, and innocence were highlighted.[70] While this focus worked, in the sense that it provided families with remission letters and a return of the confiscated goods, it did not exculpate the suicide completely. In an attempt to fully remove the stigma of suicide, many letter composers tried to establish that the suicide was not in his or her right mind when he or she died. Others went even further, arguing that the person had been under the watchful gaze of family members or neighbors, and that it was through cunning that he or she escaped from notice long enough to perform the suicidal act. For example, in 1421 Denis Sensigaut, a baker living in Saint-Marcel les Paris, had been ill for fifteen days of a 'sickness of heat'. According to the letter composed on behalf of his widow, Jehannette, he had received last rites before falling into a 'frenzy'. One day, when Denis had asked Jehannette to go to Paris to take his urine to a physician, he sent his nephew off to find him some milk and told the woman taking care of him to eat something. Having disposed of all his guards, Denis 'either by temptation of the enemy or as a result of the said frenzy and malady hung himself' by a cord he had tied to a stair in his house.[71]

As with murder, suicidal actions taken by mad people were not considered to be characteristic. Thus, madness could be imagined as a second level of exoneration. Remission rhetorically erased the crime in the eyes of the government and, at least in theory, in the eyes of the community. Remission for an action during an episode of madness might further exonerate the individual in question, since the disease in addition to the letter erased the crime from the identity. This type of erasure was easier with a suicide than with a person who was still living, since there could be no serious repercussions to making a false claim of madness in the case of suicides.[72]

69 Cohen 1993, pp. 141–142.

70 See JJ 115 fo 82 no 172; JJ 173 fo 199 no 413; and JJ 174 fo 138v no 318.

71 AN JJ 171 fo 244v no 429, edited in Longnon 1878, p. 19: 'maladie des chaleurs'; 'se soit tant par temptacion de l'ennemi comme à l'ocasion de ladite frenoisie et maladie pendu'.

72 Alexander Murray, who also examined remission letters for suicides, has suggested that these claims of madness might be questionable in such cases. Murray seems to miss the point of

Indeed, there may have been a tacit agreement within local communities that surviving relatives should not be punished for these crimes.[73] However, the question of whether or not the individual was 'really' mad is not pertinent. Rather, the fact that composers chose to understand these crimes in terms of madness means it was a plausible narrative and that people could accept the label in the context in which it was presented. Indeed, because suicide was thought of as murder of oneself, the act was directly related to those murders of family members that were equally difficult to comprehend in normal terms.[74]

Infanticide of Legitimate Children

The excuse of madness was not required as an explanation for an infanticide case to be pardoned. However, some women's families claimed they were mad when they killed their babies.[75] Generally such letters, like the letters about murder, were for particularly unusual types of infanticide, suggesting that these were more difficult cases to accept and integrate into a comprehendible narrative. There was a pattern of apparently acceptable and understandable infanticide. In these cases, women who were unmarried and generally poor became pregnant and had the baby, often while alone in their houses. These letters emphasized a number of fears that the new

letters of remission. He claims that a 'Letter of Remission, by definition, declared its beneficiary not guilty. Issued on a suicide's behalf it must prove he was not a suicide. So these letters should, in principle, be no exception to the obscurity intrinsic to suicide in French legal documents'. The trouble with his analysis lies in his insistence that remission letters were for people who were 'not guilty'. This was certainly not the case, since remission letters were in fact precisely for people who were guilty, but could be forgiven for their crime through the overarching grace of the French king. See Murray 1998, pp. 207–218.

73 Sara Butler suggests this might have also been true in English jury cases. See Butler 2006, pp. 268–275.

74 By 1450, remission for suicide had been phased out, regardless of whether the suicide was mad, suggesting either a more stringent attitude towards suicides on the part of the crown or less legal intervention on a local level. Diane Owen Hughes suggested this change in attitude might be due to humanism, which had a large contingent among the royal notaries and others in the legal profession. The humanist reading of the suicide of Lucretia was far more sympathetic than earlier Christian readings (personal communication). If so, this would suggest that the persecution of suicides fell off, rather than that it became more difficult to receive remission for such an act, but it would require considerably more research to substantiate any such assertion.

75 Remission for infanticide makes up 0.3% of Gauvard's study of crime in all remission letters, but as with suicide, it was more common as a crime committed by the mad, making up 3% of the total. Gauvard 1991, vol. 1, p. 242, table 8. For more on infanticide, see also Brissaud 1962. John Boswell 1988 suggests that people were more likely to abandon children than to kill them.

mother experienced, including the anger of parents, an inability to care for the child, and the shame of being an unwed mother. Often the woman narrated her lack of knowledge of what to do with a newborn infant as the cause of the baby's death. These narratives are fascinating for the glimpse they provide of a certain level of understanding of and compassion for these women that was not recorded in the law codes. Infanticide was viewed as a capital crime, but clearly there were exceptions to this stringent rule that took into account the economic and social problems of poor young women.[76]

The women described as mad in letters about infanticide do not fit neatly into this category of poor, unmarried, or widowed women. Rather, these were often married women with other children whose decision to kill their babies appeared inexplicable to their family and relatives. In addition, in most cases attributed to madness the child was not a newborn. The letter for Jehannette Voidié, discussed in detail in Chapter Three, represented her as a married woman with several children, who feared that her husband could not support another child. She killed the baby while taking him on a pilgrimage, when he was already several months old.[77] The disparity between this case and that of a young, unmarried mother, whose baby died within hours of birth, is clear.

These two narrative models of the poor unmarried woman and the mad woman were not mutually exclusive. It was possible to imagine poverty and the shame of an illegitimate child combining to drive a woman out of her senses. A letter composed for Michelle Galande explained that her father died when she was eight, leaving Michelle and her mother destitute. To support herself and her mother, Michelle Galande sought alms, but ten years later, as an eighteen-year-old woman, she began to be solicited by 'some' to abandon herself, which 'because of her simplicity, ignorance, and the poverty and misery in which she lived' she did, and ended up pregnant. In the end, the composers of her letter explained, it was through her fear of dishonor and shame that she 'was therefore deprived of sense and understanding' and chose to bury the baby alive rather than admit she had given birth.[78]

Infanticide was an especially disruptive crime. Women's roles were often bound up in expectations of wifehood and motherhood, confirmed

76 I have traced the development of an 'acceptable' narrative of infanticide in this period, which I intend to make the focus of further study. For more on this development, and on a parallel shift in the thinking of the theologian Jean Gerson, who called for a more mild penitence in cases of accidental infanticide, see Gauvard and Ouy 2001.

77 AN JJ 172 fo 239 no 430, edited in Longnon 1878, pp. 130–133.

78 AN JJ 221 fo 30 no 35: 'par sa simplesse et ignorance et la povrete et misere en quoy elle estoit'; 'estoit lors despournent de sens et entendement'.

through the idealized figure of the Virgin Mary.[79] The murder of a helpless baby ruptured expectations of safety and comfort, and the mother's role as murderer, rather than protector, highlighted the enormity of the act. Infanticide can be seen as an extreme version of the larger pattern of mad murders that violated the idealized image of the peaceful interior of familial relationships. While some forms of infanticide by poor, young, and unmarried girls, might be comprehensible, the killing of a legitimate baby was not.

Bestiality

Whereas infanticide was a crime that was gendered female, bestiality was a crime that was gendered male.[80] Like the other crimes examined here, it was possible to gain remission for bestiality without claiming to have been mad, but occasionally the letters include madness as an explanatory device. Bestiality was another crime against the self, the family, and the community, since it was a sexual act removed from the appropriate venue of the marriage bed. Much like infanticide, bestiality appears to have a conventional narrative, even though it appeared much less frequently in the remission letters. This narrative focused on the youth and unmarried status of the perpetrator, in much the same way as letters for infanticide. Generally the young man was described as a teenager, and the crime usually took place alone, most often with the mare that was pulling his cart, a sheep he was guarding, or a cow in the stables.

Estienne Perdereau's remission letter from 1481 told a fascinating tale of how youthful mistakes could come back to haunt a person later in life. According to his narrative, when he was thirteen or fourteen (around sixteen or seventeen years previously, as he was about thirty when he sought remission, and the perfect age to commit a crime, since he was on the border of adulthood and could not be held legally responsible[81]), he had taken a cart into the woods, pulled by a mare. While there, he was tempted by the 'enemy from hell' into trying to have 'carnal company' with the mare, since he had not yet had 'carnal company' with a woman.[82] However, before he could achieve his 'evil desire', he saw Guillot Baillif, a neighbor of his master's, and

79 Indeed, other idealized mother figures in medieval religious art included the mothers who tried to protect their children in images of the massacre of the Holy Innocents. Presciutti 2015, p. 168; see also Presciutti 2011.

80 Strangely, although the first bestiality case I found dates from 1406, well within the range of Gauvard's study, she does not mention it in her own analysis of the letters.

81 The age of adulthood was fourteen for boys and twelve for girls.

82 AN JJ 209 fo 93v no 170: 'tempte de lennemi denfer'; 'compaignie charnelle'.

'as soon as he saw the said Guillot he returned to his good memory'.[83] Thus, Estienne had been out of his 'good memory', and therefore was associating his mental state with madness, when he attempted to have sex with the mare. Not only did Estienne never consummate his bestial temptation, as he explained, but he immediately went to the church of Notre Dame de Clery and confessed his sinful desire to a priest, who absolved him and gave him a penance that he completed 'as well as he could'.[84] Estienne proceeded to get married and live an exemplary life until one day, as he explained, he refused to give a pair of shoes to Guillot Baillif, who conceived such a great hatred for Estienne that he accused him of bestiality to the local justice and had him thrown in prison. As Estienne took pains to demonstrate, his actions were not, in the end, damaging to himself, to the mare, or to the community. He 'returned to his good memory' before taking the ultimate step, immediately reconciled himself with the church, and a few years later married and became a respectable member of the community. Guillot Baillif, rather, appeared unsavory in Estienne's narrative, waiting for seventeen years before bringing the case to the attention of the local justice due to a grudge.

The question of who would be harmed by bestiality was addressed obliquely in another case. In 1406, the seventeen-year-old Piot le Pele had been living for a year as a servant of the family of Piot Pichon, during which time he slept in the stable with the cows. Note that, at seventeen, Piot le Pele was too old to be considered a child, and therefore would be held accountable for his actions. Instead, the letter noted immediately that Piot le Pele was 'mad and out of all memory'.[85] He 'was tempted by the enemy combined with his insensibility such that he had carnal company and habitation with this cow'.[86] Significantly, it was his mistress and her daughters who saw him do this and spread the gossip around the community, highlighting the dangers of bestiality as a crime against the community. The unmarried daughters of Piot Pichon were troubled by the actions of Piot le Pele. Indeed, perhaps it would have been more easily reconciled had he sought sexual release from one of them. After all, confession manuals saw fornication as a less problematic sexual sin, and some city governments in Italy explained

83 AN JJ 209 fo 93v no 170: 'mauvaise voulenter'; 'incontinant quil apperceut ledit guillot revien a son bon memoire'.

84 AN JJ 209 fo 93v no 170: 'au mieulx quil a peu'.

85 AN JJ 160 fo 264v no 372: 'fol et hors de toute memoire'.

86 AN JJ 160 fo 264v no 372: 'fu tempte par lennemy avec son insensibilite quil ot compaignie et habitacion charnelle a ycelle vache'.

their decision to allow prostitution by justifying it as an alternative to other types of sexual deviance.[87]

In both of these cases, the men were young and had not yet had 'carnal company' with a woman. Their status as unmarried youths made their sexual crime less dangerous, but they were still threatening the morality of the community. The narratives of their remission letters turned attention to the questionable actions of their accusers. Guillot Baillif did not register a complaint until he had another reason to be angry with Estienne Perdereau. Indeed, Estienne, whose madness was temporary and did not even lead to the consummation of his misplaced desire, had confessed to his sinful thoughts immediately, going through the appropriate channel of the parish priest. Similarly, Piot le Pele, who was known to be 'fol', was witnessed by the women of the household, who chose to gossip about him in the community, thus spreading the problem further. Unlike Estienne, Piot did not seek out confession, and he had carried through with his desire. However, Piot's madness was not described as a temporary state, but as a long-term problem.

Arson

According to the customary law books of Normandy, mad people must be kept chained up or under guard specifically to prevent them from setting fires.[88] Interestingly, although this seems to be a perceived danger in general terms, it appears in only nine remission letters as a crime committed by mad people. Sometimes the letters merely described the arsonist in question as 'simple' or out of their senses due to excessive drunkenness, but occasionally fires were set by people who are described as emphatically out of their minds. Again, the crime appeared particularly troublesome because it attacked the community the mad person ought to defend. Indeed, some of the narratives were about people setting fire to their own homes or barns. This particular crime highlighted the fear of mad people as disruptive members of the community, since fires in medieval villages (especially in regions where wood and wattle were used as building materials) would have been highly damaging and uncontrollable.

In 1379, for example, Guille de la Barre, a wealthy man, began to suffer a reversal of fortune. He lost so much that he 'had displeasure in his life and

87 Brundage 1987; Hughes 2004, p. 114; Trexler 1981.
88 Gruchy 1881, p. 184, LXXIX.

wanted very much to be dead'.[89] However, it was at the moment when a court case was decided against him that Guille 'entered into a sickness such that he became totally altered and completely thus as if completely out of his senses' and began to say that God did not love him, since He allowed such terrible things to happen to him.[90] In his despair, Guille lit two of the beds in his own home on fire. Fortunately, the local officers of justice were apprised of the situation before too much damage was done. The extremity of Guille's actions was highlighted by his statement blaming God for his misfortune. His wanton destruction that threatened the entire town stemmed from his altered state, in which he could not be held responsible for his actions.

In some cases, arson attacks were not targeted at the person's own goods. One case in particular stands out for its complex narrative leading up to the fire. In 1427, Jahenne de la Boronne, wife of Guillaume and mother of four small children, including one who was only a month old, left her home to run some errands. The letter explains that she was 'light-headed', and 'stayed a long time'. When she returned home, her husband asked why she had left for so long, such that her youngest child was in a 'bad state'. Jehanne replied angrily that it was at the request of Estiennote, wife of Martin Raccavel, who she believed was having an affair with Guillaume. Seeing Estiennote nearby, Jehanne began to verbally attack her, asking 'why she had been false to her husband'. The two women began arguing with each other until Guillaume intervened, taking Jehanne home and beating her until she 'was calm enough'. He then left the house to tend their animals, at which point Jehanne, who was apparently not calm enough yet, 'left the said house as if completely despairing and out of her good senses' and burned down a house belonging to Estiennote that was worth six livres tournois.[91] This is simultaneously a typical narrative about jealousy and spousal infidelity and a shocking story about the actions of a woman who is out of her mind. Much like some of the suicide narratives discussed above, this letter exculpates Jehanne on multiple levels. Though her anger and despair about her husband cheating on her with their neighbor was understandable, her response was disproportionate and could only be explained if she were mad at the time.

89 AN JJ 115 fo 34 no 75: 'a eu desplaisance de sa vie et voulsist bien estre mort'.

90 AN JJ 115 fo 34 no 75: 'entra en une maladie telement que il devint tout altere et tout ainsi comme tout hors du sens'.

91 AN JJ 174 fo 7 no 17: 'legier de teste'; 'longuement demouree'; 'mauvais estat'; 'pour quoy elle lui avoit forfait son mary'; 'fu assez apaisee'; 'se parti dudit hostel comme toutes desesperee ou hors de son bon sens'.

Mad Victims of Crime

Mad people did not only appear in remission letters as the central figure of the criminal. Indeed, often they appeared as the victims of murder, who had to be killed because their madness threatened the lives of others. In many of these cases, they were perceived not as individuals who could be returned to their 'good reputation', but rather as dangerously and frighteningly uncontrollable potential criminals. However, sometimes (especially when they were related to their killers) they were simultaneously described as unfortunate victims of their madness.

Several letters involving mad victims follow a typical pattern of describing a bar brawl, explaining that the people involved had been drinking and eating before the violence broke out. Drunkenness was seen as exacerbating or even causing madness in these cases, and the letters describe a fight that was forced to turn deadly because of the victim's lack of sense or understanding.[92] According to these narratives, the mad were generally unpleasant people whose moments of madness were merely another negative aspect of their personalities.

A slightly more complicated narrative about a mad victim comes from a remission for Jehan Mondit in 1490. A mason, Jehan Mondit had been hired by Christophe Asse, seigneur de Rollière, counselor and chamberlain of King Charles VIII, to build a chapel in La Rollière, a small town near Parthenay. While he was living there, he got to know a certain Cappitaine Trigalle, 'a man of little understanding known as a fool'. One Friday evening, after eating and drinking in Parthenay, Trigalle arrived back in La Rollière where Christophe Asse and his men began to mock him and dance with him, laughing and exchanging 'joyous words'. Afterwards, the seigneur commanded his men to go to bed, leaving Trigalle alone. When Jehan Mondit returned to the courtyard alone, planning to go to bed, he saw Trigalle leaving the house, carrying a naked sword in both hands. Trigalle came running up to Jehan, 'swearing on the blood and the mother of Our Lord that he would kill him'. Jehan responded that he had no quarrel with Trigalle, and the mad man left him and ran towards the bridge, where he found Jehan Mondit's varlet and began again to swear and menace this new target. At this point, 'hearing the sound and the noise, knowing that the said Trigalle was mad and dangerous as truly he was', Jehan Mondit went to his varlet's aid, pulling the attention of Trigalle, who did not recognize

92 See AN JJ 172 fo 113v no 221 (in 1422); AN JJ 181 fo 19 no 30 (in 1451); AN JJ 219 fo 132 no 216 (in 1488).

him and was still armed with a sword. Trigalle managed to wound Jehan Mondit before he was finally able to get in a single hit on Trigalle's temple. Too late, Christophe Asse and his men arrived on the scene and took Trigalle back to the house, where the next day he died.[93] This narrative gives us access to a moment when mockery of a reputed 'fool' went horribly awry. Jehan Mondit, who does not appear to have participated in the earlier raillery, is threatened nevertheless by the mad man. Trigalle appears as an amusing and entertaining fool early in the letter, then an uncontrollable blasphemer running around with a naked sword, unable to understand what he is doing.[94]

Even the murdered mad could appear as victims when they were family members rather than strangers, however. Just as mad people murdered family members because of their uncontrollable actions, so they could drive their family to kill them with the same behaviors. Around the year 1362, Margueroy la Marchande moved into the home of her nephew, Jehan Langlois, because she could not take care of herself.[95] It appears that she may have disagreed with that assessment, since according to the letter composed on behalf of Jehan Langlois, she tried to run away several times but he always brought her back. The letter explains that she ran away due to her 'foolish and simple desire and without any cause'.[96] Finally, when she got up at two in the morning and left the house, Jehan followed her,

93 AN JJ 221 fo 32 no 39: 'homme de petit entendement repute comme fol'; 'joyeuses parolles'; 'juroit le sang et la mere de notre sieur quil le tueroit'; 'ouyt le bruit et la noyse sachant que ledit trigalle este fol et dangereux comme ala verite si este'.

94 It is unclear whether Trigalle was employed by Christophe Asse, but he does seem to fulfil a similar function to a court fool. The idea that fools employed by nobles could become violent and even that their violence could be part of their amusement value appears in Pierre de Fenin's memoires from the year 1423. In this incident, a number of fools were given twelve gold pieces. They put each gold piece in a large, silver drinking cup and then filled the cups with wine, saying whoever drank the wine should have the gold piece in it. Dalleret, the fool of Count Valeran of Saint-Pol, decided he would drink all twelve cups and have all twelve pieces of gold and proceeded to do so. When the other fools realized they had lost all their gold, they attacked Dalleret and beat him until he died. Fenin notes: 'for this reason we ridiculed them greatly' ('on fist mainte risée pour ceste besoingne'). Pierre de Fenin 1837, p. 202.

95 Whereas the Roman practice gave guardians to all mad people, French customals usually assigned guardians only to those insane from birth. Philippe de Beaumanoir used clear language to distinguish between these two different types of mad people, and it was only the *fous de nature*, those mad from birth, who were to be assigned guardians. Philippe de Beaumanoir 1970–1974, vol. 2, ch. 56, paragraph 1624. The *Livres de jostice* established similar rules for protecting the rights and privileges of the mad by placing them in the care of a guardian. Rapetti 1850, p. 59, IX.5. These customals assigned wardship to the relatives of the mad to deal with the complicated question of inheritance. See Pfau 2008, Chapter 2 and Ternon 2018.

96 AN JJ 99 fo 33 no 104: 'desa volonte fols et simple et sens aucune cas raison'.

reportedly because he feared she would commit suicide by drowning herself in a fosse (a ditch or moat generally filled with water) or a well. He caught up with her next to a large fosse full of water and tried to take her home, but when she refused, he angrily hit her with a little stick four or five times, 'without blood and without wound and without doing anything else to her from which she might become ill nor have death come to her'.[97] Regardless of how minor a reprimand he gave her, Jehan's aunt died about fifteen days later, and five years after that he and his wife and children sought remission for this act. Marguerey was not actively threatening anyone but herself, but her actions were inexplicable to her nephew and he used her mad behavior to justify beating her.

III. Proofs of Madness

In addition to representing the crimes committed by mad people as particularly damaging to their communal identity, many letters highlighted previous acts that indicated the person was mad to provide proof of madness. Not all letters indicate how long the individual was considered mad by others, but those that do range from a lifetime to the moments before the crime. The common medieval belief that mad behavior was instantly recognizable and, indeed, easily replicable by the sane, is significant for thinking about the meaning of madness in criminal cases. There were many ways to describe madness, but each one sought to provide proof, not only that the individual was unquestionably behaving as a mad person would, but also that this madness was either a long-standing issue in his or her life or a clear and real disturbance, not merely enacted conveniently at the moment of the crime. Because madness was acknowledged as imitable behavior, many of the letters provide case histories demonstrating that this was not a case of simulation. In doing so, they were responding to concerns expressed in both religious and legal discourse about the possibility of counterfeiting madness.

In the Bible, the ability to feign madness was represented as a positive way to avoid punishment. The event occurred during Saul's reign, after God had chosen David as the new king of Israel and sent an evil spirit to trouble Saul, who remained on the throne. Jealous of David, Saul attempted to have him killed, and David was forced into exile in the kingdom of Geth.

97 AN JJ 99 fo 33 no 104: 'sanz sang et sens plaie et sens autre mal luy fait dont elle deust estre malade ne mort ensuivant en sa personne'.

In this case David used gestures coded as madness to fool his enemies into ignoring him, thus allowing him to escape:

> And the servants of Achis, when they saw David, said to him: Is not this David the king of the land? Did they not sing to him in their dances, saying: Saul hath slain his thousands, and David his ten thousands? But David laid up these words in his heart, and was exceedingly afraid at the face of Achis the king of Geth. And he changed his countenance before them, and slipt down between their hands: and he stumbled against the doors of the gate, and his spittle ran down upon his beard. And Achis said to his servants: You saw the man was mad: why have you brought him to me? Have we need of madmen, that you have brought in this fellow, to play the madman in my presence? Shall this fellow come into my house?[98]

David's behavior demonstrates the ease with which madness could be copied. He merely stumbled and drooled on himself, and his enemies immediately interpreted him as 'insane' and 'furious', to give more accurate translations than the Douay-Rheims Bible provides. While in this case David's deceit allows him to escape an inappropriate punishment by a king who had lost God's favor, the Bible affirms the potential ease with which madness could be performed by the sane.

In his *Coutumes de Beauvaisis*, Philippe de Beaumanoir expressed concerns about the possibility that the accused could pretend to be mad in order to avoid legitimate punishment. This question would most likely arise, according to Philippe de Beaumanoir, when a mad person was perceived to have recovered from his or her madness and was released, at which point

> one should examine considerably whether this was not done maliciously, for example if some people, when they had committed offenses, counterfeited being out of their senses [*le hors du sens*] in order to escape: and one should regard very closely what cause motivated the person

98 First Book of Kings 21:11–15. 'dixeruntque ei servi Achis numquid non iste est David rex terrae nonne huic cantabant per choros dicentes percussit Saul mille et David decem milia posuit autem David sermones istos in corde suo et extimuit valde a facie Achis regis Geth et inmutavit os suum coram eis et conlabebatur inter manus eorum et inpingebat in ostia portae defluebantque salivae eius in barbam et ait Achis ad servos suos vidistis hominem insanum quare adduxistis eum ad me an desunt nobis furiosi quod introduxistis istum ut fureret me praesente hicine ingredietur domum meam'.

> to commit the misdeed, and by this one will know if there was deceit [*barat*].[99]

This fear of *barat*, which can be translated as a fraud, a deception, or a ruse, was querying the concept that madness was, in fact, a transparent phenomenon, and posed the theory that a person could imitate madness to avoid being punished for a real criminal act. For Philippe de Beaumanoir, the proof of madness would come from a close examination of what 'moved' the criminal, suggesting that a sane criminal would have different motivations than a mad criminal. According to this conception of madness, witnesses would not be able to tell from a person's actions whether or not he or she was mad. Instead, it would be necessary to consider the motives for the act to see whether or not the act itself was done due to madness.

Similarly, the author of the *Livres de jostice*, aware of the conception of madness as a cyclical disease, insisted that mad people who committed their crimes during a period of sanity should not go unpunished. According to the book,

> the king says that it is necessary to take care with a mad person [*desvé*] who kills his father, whether he had done it in good sense or in madness [*desverie*]; and if he did it in good sense, he must pay for it. – And if you know certainly that he did it in madness [*forsenerie*], that he does not know what he does every day, and that he understands nothing, nor is there any suspicion against him, you can in a way cut his sentence, because he is tormented enough by his madness [*desverie*]: and he must always be well guarded [...]. And if it happens, as it sometimes does, that someone is mad [*desvé*] at one time and at other times is sane, and was sane at the moment when he did the deed, you should enquire diligently; and if you know it, you will not pardon him; and if it happens that you know that he did it by felony, it is right that he be tormented.[100]

99 Philippe de Beaumanoir 1970–1974, vol. 2, ch. 52, paragraph 1575: 'Et s'il revient bien en son sens, il doit estre delivrés de prison, et li siens rendus. Mes en ce cas se doit l'en mout regarder que ce ne soit fet malicieusement, si comme li aucun, quant il avroient fet les mesfès, contreferoient le hors du sens pour eschaper: si doit l'en mout regarder quele cause le mut a fere le mesfet et par ce savra l'en s'il i a barat'.

100 Rapetti 1850, p. 73 XXI.5: 'Et se l'en ne puet tenir aucun desvé, il doivent metre aucun consel et remède qu'il soient mis en prison, et issint le commende li rois. Et li rois dit que l'en se devoit prendre garde au desvé qui tue son père, s'il l'avet fet en bon sen ou en desverie; et s'il l'avet fet en bon sen, il le doit comparer. -- Et se tu sés certainement que il l'ait fet en forsenerie, qu'il ne sache qu'il face toz jorz, et qu'il n'entende riens, n'en i ait point de sopeçon contre lui, tu porras en une feintise estramper sa paine, quar il est assez tormentez de sa desverie: et totes voies le

The author of the *Livres de jostice* took great care to distinguish between those who commit a crime while mad and those who commit a crime in 'good sense'. Unfortunately, there is no indication of how to 'know certainly' nor from whom one should 'enquire diligently' to 'know' that the mad person was sane at the moment of the act. It is likely that the question would have been directed to any witnesses of the crime, suggesting that, for the author of the *Livres de jostice*, madness was an externally recognizable state that could be judged by any witness. Knowledge of an individual's mental state would be difficult to prove beyond doubt, but a description of the person's performance of the criminal act could establish sanity or insanity.

Some letters sought to prove a person's madness simply by establishing that the condition had been recognized for a long time. So, for example, in 1378 the fifteen-year-old Jachete le Pernec was described as being 'of small understanding and natural sense' for her whole life before burning down her home in response to a dispute with a woman who lived with her.[101] Similarly, Pierre Chambo 'called le Fol' was described as having always been 'like a complete idiot without having sense or discretion' when he got into an argument about paying the bill at a tavern in 1390 and ended up killing Pierre Audrieu.[102] In these cases, madness was simply a part of the individual's identity, even becoming Pierre Chambo's nickname, and the composers of these letters saw no need to explain further how they knew these people were mad.

On the other extreme, some letters described a temporary madness that overtook the person for the moments before the crime and then disappeared. So, for example, in a 1489 letter about infanticide discussed in more detail above, the relatives of Michelle Galande explained that when she gave birth, she 'was for the moment deprived of sense and understanding' and buried her baby alive in a ditch.[103] Another case of temporary madness had a clear external cause. Clement Marie took care of his seventy-year-old uncle Michiel who was unable to walk. One evening they got into an argument and Michiel hit Clement over the head with a stick, stunning him so that he did not know what he was doing when he hit his uncle back, giving Michiel a

doit l'en bien garder [...]. Et s'il avient, comme aucunes foiz, que aucuns sunt desvé une foiz et autre foiz sont sein, et fust seins en celui point où il fit le fait, tu l'enquerras diligement; et se tu le sés, tu ne li pardonras pas; et s'il est issit que tu saches qu'il l'ait fait par félonie, droiz est qu'il soit tormentez'.

101 AN JJ 114 fo 70v no 147: 'de petite cognoissance et senz naturel'.

102 AN JJ 140 fo 83 no 67: 'comme tout ydiote non aiant senz ne discrettion'.

103 AN JJ 221 fo 30 no 35: 'estoit lors despournent de sens et entendement'.

wound from which he later died.[104] In 1364, a temporary madness overcame Jehan Razochez, a baker who was angered by the taxes he had to pay. His anger was so intense that he was described as 'maddened by grief' when he blasphemed in front of the town's mayor.[105] These cases of temporary madness also required no further explanation and relied on the extremity of the moment described to prove the person was truly mad.

When the madness was neither lifelong nor momentary, letter composers often chose to describe previous episodes of what they considered mad behavior in order to provide proof that the madness was real. Some relied on behaviors universally acknowledged to be unacceptable to create a pattern of madness that would be easily recognizable as inappropriate without elucidating the individual's patterns of behavior before becoming mad. Attempted suicide is one of the most commonly used referents in these cases. These were almost always efforts to throw oneself into a well or a ditch to drown. To list a few cases already described above, Pierre de Solente's family feared he would commit suicide, and after he killed his son his wife found him attempting to drown himself in a river.[106] Similarly, Ysabeau, daughter of Raymon Sarvallier, tried to throw herself into two different wells around town, including one at a convent.[107] Margueroy la Marchande's nephew feared she would drown herself in a fosse or a well, though it is unclear whether she actually had that intention.[108] Jehanne, the wife of Chrestien Bolu, decided to drown herself and her children in a small river at the bottom of her garden, though in the end she only drowned one of them.[109] Jehan le Vignon attempted to throw himself in a well and kill himself, but his wife (whom he later murdered) prevented it.[110]

The story of Marion, wife of Jehan de Fresnes, drives home the link between suicide attempts and behavior that threatens the family. In 1415, Marion who 'previously had been harmed in the brain [...] and previously had been tempted to drown herself' sent her six-year-old daughter to the solar with an apple then followed her up the ladder with a cord and a knife. When she arrived, in a parody of motherly concern, she asked her daughter what

104 AN JJ 131 fo 39v no 69.

105 AN JJ 98 fo 36v no 113: 'forcenez de grief'. The next chapter considers in more detail the ways extreme emotions were understood in terms of madness to provide space for the resolution of disruptions in the family and community.

106 AN JJ 110 fo 125 no 108.

107 AN JJ 163 fo 130 no 229.

108 AN JJ 99 fo 33 no 104.

109 AN JJ 195 fo 268v no 1204.

110 AN JJ 78 fo 145 no 262.

she had in her throat. Her daughter replied that it was a piece of the apple she had eaten. Marion asked her to show it to her, and when her daughter did, Marion grabbed her and cut her throat with the knife. Afterwards, she used the cord to create a noose and tried to hang herself. However, there was a bale of straw underneath her on which she placed a foot and began to call for help. Two neighbor women arrived and found Marion and her daughter.[111] Marion's earlier attempts to kill herself provide context for understanding her murderous attack on her daughter.

Another case also demonstrates this link. Jacquet Morniet had been ill for a time when he killed his brother's wife Jehanne, who lived with him and his brother in their extended household along with their parents and children. After picking up a pestle and hitting her over the head, Jacquet ran out of the house 'wishing and attempting to go throw and drown himself in a well,' but his brother stopped him.[112] In this case, Jacquet's suicide attempt emerged after he had already committed a terrible crime that disrupted his household. Perhaps because suicide was viewed as such a departure from acceptable behavior, it could be used as a clear indication of madness.

Nakedness and running through the fields were also considered general behavioral signs of madness. Pierre de Solente ran out of his house 'completely naked' after killing his son.[113] Jehan Massetirer also 'got up from his bed completely naked' and fled the house to throw himself in a well.[114] Jehan Cavrignon also got up from his bed 'completely naked being in his chemise' and set fire to his father's home and outbuildings.[115] In some ways, this concept drew from medieval literary depictions of madness. The idealized chivalric knight in French literature is constantly engaged in a performance of his identity, according to Susan Crane.[116] In madness, these performances of civilized identity are transformed into performances of bestial savagery. Yvain, for example, is driven mad by the loss of his lady's love.[117] Yvain reverts to animalistic behavior, living naked in the woods and eating meat raw. His behavior is the extreme antithesis of ideal courtly behavior, and he is

111 AN JJ 169 fo 17 no 26: 'autrefoiz avoit este blecee ou cerveil […] et dont autreffoiz elle avoit este temptee de soy noyer'.

112 AN JJ 188 fo 102 no 203: 'voulant et tendent a soy aler gecter et noyer en ung puiz'.

113 AN JJ 110 fo 125 no 108: 'tout nu'.

114 AN JJ 146 fo 65 no 129: 'il se leva de son lit tout nu'.

115 AN JJ 204 fo 6v no 13: 'tout nu estans en son chemise'.

116 Crane 2002, pp. 107–139.

117 Chrétien de Troyes 1994, p. 274. Lines 2805–2809: 'El chief, si grant quë il forsenne;/Lors se desschire et se despenne/Et fuit par cans et par valees,/Si laisse ses gens esgarees,/Qu'il se merveillent ou puet ester'.

only recognizable through the scars on his body that indicate his former status as a knight who fought battles and won tournaments.[118] This loss of love leading to loss of sanity and a reversion to bestial behavior became a common pattern in later romances.[119] The image of the relationship between insanity and bestial behavior, or of madness as a return to nature, made a clear connection between wildmen and the mad people in romances who, through losing their senses, lose their civility. Joyce Salisbury notes that wildmen fulfilled a particular function in medieval thought, arguing that the 'concept of a negative human, one who embodied everything humans did not, must have presented a strangely comforting figure because it threw into focus precisely those qualities that defined humanity: rational thought, social behavior, cleanliness, clothing, etc'.[120]

Both suicide attempts and public nudity were universally recognized as disruptive and inappropriate behavior. However, many letters described much more specific, focused, and personal disruptions, as is clear from the case of Jehan de Moustier whose narrative is discussed at the opening of this chapter. Similarly, before murdering her husband, Jehannecte Troppé began exhibiting behaviors viewed as disruptive by her family and friends, destroying her household goods and scattering flour around the floor.[121] In general, in composing these letters, family and friends tended to focus on describing earlier behaviors that did not fit into their understandings of normal actions to contextualize the criminal act as an aberration.

The types of crimes committed by people described as mad, as well as the roles played by mad people as causes of crime or victims of crime, provided an image of madness as a disruption of kin and communal values and norms. The victims of mad crimes were often family members or neighbors with whom the mad person and his or her family had previously lived in harmony. The significance of the crimes committed by people who were believed to be mad lay not as much in the actual act but in the victims of those acts. Even when mad people caused a crime to occur, they were implicated in that crime specifically because of their inability to conform to expected patterns of behavior and because that inability threatened their family and community. These crimes were troubling because they disrupted accepted

118 Chrétien de Troyes 1994, pp. 280–282.

119 Mary Frances Wack has written an excellent book about medieval medical and literary ideas about lovesickness, which is distinct from (although related to) madness. See Wack 1990.

120 Salisbury 1994, p. 152. Richard Bernheimer had similarly argued that there was a 'psychological need' for a figure like the wildman in the Middle Ages. See Bernheimer 1952.

121 AN JJ 173 no 63 fo 33v. Edited in Le Cacheux 1907–1908, pp. 181–183.

social codes, not because of the nature of the crime itself, but because the victim of that crime was someone or something that should not be targeted by the mad person. These remission letters sought to tell a story that embedded the particular moment of the crime in a narrative structure that could explain these ruptures as part of a general pattern of mad behavior. It is precisely through attempts to comprehend these misconceptions of the mad that these narratives can begin to allow a reconciliation between the mad person, or the mad person's family, and the community. By trying to explain the transgressions of the mad in comprehensible terms, the narratives provided a bridge to reconnect the kin and community ties ruptured through the particularities of the mad person's crime. The family's choice to seek a remission letter to advocate for the mad person was a particularly resonant act on his or her behalf. The next chapter considers the way the very kin and communal ties that had been threatened through the actions of the mad were reaffirmed through these letters of remission.

3. Reintegrating Madness

The Mad in Their Communities

Abstract
Remission letters provide evidence for community and family actions and the networks available to help or hinder the mad. While the crimes of the mentally ill most often targeted their kin and communal ties, through the medium of remission letters, these ties were reformed, and connections were reconstructed. The family and the community simultaneously wished to aid the mad and feared the possible consequences of insanity. In some cases, the remission letters sought to tell the story from the perspective of the criminal, thereby encouraging the family members and the notary composing the letter to attempt to rationalize the insanity, creating an alternative understanding of reality through which the mad person's crime was comprehensible.

Keyterms: Reputation, Protection, Justice, Understanding

When the French king, Charles VI, had his first episode of madness in 1392, the chroniclers described an intense response by the entire realm of France. Michel Pintoin, the chronicler of Saint-Denis, explained in detail:

> [w]hen the news was spread throughout the realm, all the true French cried as if for the death of an only son; so much was the health of France attached to that of its king! The clergy, seeing that human remedies were powerless against this strange illness, called on heaven, between tears and sobs, with fervent prayers for the conservation of a life so precious. In all the churches, they added to the divine office oraisons specifically for the king. The bishops, accompanied by their clergy, made processions from church to church. Men and women followed them, barefoot, prostrating themselves before the Lord with groans

Pfau, A., *Medieval Communities and the Mad: Narratives of Crime and Mental Illness in Late Medieval France.* Taylor & Francis Group, 2021
DOI: 10.5117/9789462983359_CH03

> and tears, and asked him with one contrite and humble heart for the recovery of the king.[1]

Michel Pintoin was quick to acknowledge that this moving display of unity, with all 'true French' acting with one heart, touched God's heart and led to the king's recovery. Clearly, the chronicler felt that Charles VI's suffering needed divine aid, which could be sought through the intercession of the people of his realm. He linked 'true French' identity and prayers for the king here, 'imagining' or even re-imagining the French realm in terms of the king's madness.[2] As he continued to write about the king's cyclical illness over the next three decades, Michel Pintoin was certain the king's every recovery was due to God's pity for the prayers of the French people. Even when he was simply making a passing reference to the king's recovery, he referred to Charles' 'incolumitas', or 'safety'.[3] This Latin term was unusual in Classical Latin, but would have been easily recognizable to a medieval audience as part of the liturgy. When masses were said for the king's recovery, the French people asked for his 'salus et incolumitas'.[4] The French king's madness simultaneously threatened the cohesion of the French realm and provided an opportunity for the inhabitants of that realm to come together and reaffirm their communal identity and belonging.[5] On a much smaller scale, remission letters for mad

1 Bellaguet 1842, vol. 2, p. 22: 'Ut autem per regnum divulgatum est, omnes veri Francigene tanquam super unigenitorum morte doluerunt. Equidem omnium regnicolarum salus in sua fundata erat. Ideo viri ecclesiastici attendentes, quod vis morbi humanis subsidiis sublevari non poterat, quanto desiderio tunc ipsam affectabant, tanto fervore devocionis et cum mestis singultibus ad Deum se converterunt. Ubique certe facte fuerunt pro ipsa oraciones in celebracione divinorum ab universa Ecclesia. Episcopi cum clero arma de ecclesiis ad ecclesias bajulantes spiritualia, sexu utriusque plebis nudis vestigiis subsequente, ante Dominum prostrati, cum gemitu et lacrimis, corde contrito et humiliato, orabant pro incolumitate regis'.

2 Here I am playing with the term 'imagined community' coined by Benedict Anderson. Though Anderson argues that the printing press was necessary for the creation of an 'imagined community' on the scale of the realm, his oversimplified vision of the Middle Ages suggests that medieval Christians 'had no conception of history as an end-less chain of cause and effect or of radical separations between past and present' and thus were incapable of 'thinking a nation'. Anderson 1983, pp. 23–36. This view has been challenged by medievalists. See especially the essays collected in Forde, Johnson, and Murray 1995. As I have argued elsewhere, the French realm was 'imagined' and constructed just as much as the later nation has been. Pfau 2008, p. 52.

3 Bellaguet 1842, vol. 2, p. 22.

4 Boyle, Byler, and Halsall 1996: 'pro spe salutis, et incolumitis suae'.

5 As others have argued, processions symbolically represented the body politic by enacting and displaying social roles and hierarchies. It is important to remember the inhabitants themselves performed these spectacles, inscribing their own location within the community through the act of walking the town in which they resided, or through the experience of viewing others moving through space. Spectators were just as much part of the procession as those who were actively

criminals operated in the same way. These letters construed mad crimes as acts that disrupted a person's social identity, which was defined through kin and communal bonds. Nevertheless, by their very nature, these letters sought to reintegrate the mad criminal into their community.

Just as the processions undertaken on behalf of the French king's health sought to deny and suppress the very real fissures in the body politic to present a unified 'true France', the composers of remission letters for the mad drew on idealized visions of communal responsibility in their texts. In doing so, they created an 'imagined community' that differed significantly from the one in which they actually lived, and tied these supplicants and their local communities to the larger French realm, where the king heard their individual complaints and repaired their damaged communities. The letters inscribed an image of a cohesive community ruptured by the madness of the individual. Despite or perhaps even because of this rupture, the communities envisioned by the letter composers worked towards resolution and restructuring. They reimagined the past by exploring options for preventing the crimes of the mad before they occurred, and suggested hopes for the future by reintegrating the mad into their families and communities. When the madness was purportedly of long standing, these letters included details about attempts made to cure the mad by taking them on pilgrimages or, in one case, seeking a physician's aid. The letters also described methods of restraining the mad, by keeping them in chains, or locking them in a small room or outbuilding. Some were kept under surveillance, guarded by their family or by helpful neighbors. These recollections of seeking cures for the mad or attempting to guard them placed the concerns of the mad at the center of the families' prayers and daily lives.

I. Reputation and Renown

One of the most significant goals of all remission letters was the restoration of the individual's reputation. While all pardon recipients were returned to their previous 'good reputation', the discourse of madness allowed for an even stronger claim that the crime committed did not fit within the character of the perpetrator. For example, in a letter written on behalf of Jehannecte de la Forge, a widow living in Saint Germain la Ville, the composers explained that she had been 'often mad and deprived of reasonable understanding and

moving. For more on processions, see Guenée 2004, p. 174; Guenée 1999, pp. 23–49; Guenée and Lehoux 1968; Flanigan 2001, p. 39; Fassler 2007, pp. 13–62.

of all sense'.[6] She was taken to Notre Dame de Tanovay in 1403, presumably seeking a cure, though the letter does not specify that. One day she was walking down the street when she came across her granddaughter, who was about eighteen months old, 'whom she loved as much as she could when she was in her good senses'.[7] In her madness, however, she threw the child to the ground and cut her throat with a 'scipe' (perhaps a scissor) and killed her. The letter emphasized that Jehannecte de la Forge 'had never had any hatred for her or for any relatives of hers'.[8] Clearly, the actions of Jehannecte de la Forge when mad were a departure from her identity when sane. The murder of a young child whom she loved when she was sane was only explicable in the context of her lack of sense. The composers of her letter of remission fulfilled a dual purpose in commenting that she had no quarrel with the girl or with her family. This statement simultaneously denied the possibility that the murder might have been motivated by some familial rivalry and insisted on the disconnection between Jehannecte de la Forge's status as a widow in the community and her actions while mad. The formula at the end of her letter, similar to all others, reads:

> we acquit, remit, and pardon in the abovesaid case by our special grace and royal authority the deed and case abovesaid with all penalty, offence, and fine corporal, criminal, and civil which by rigor of justice she could incur against us, and we restore her to her good reputation and renown in the country and to her unconfiscated goods, and on this [subject] we impose perpetual silence on our procurer.[9]

Despite Jehannecte de la Forge's madness that caused her to murder her own daughter's daughter, the king promised to restore her to her good reputation and impose perpetual silence on the subject. In a moment of cognitive tension, the letter sought to erase the crime by telling the full story of it publicly and openly.

6 AN JJ 158 fo 11 no 20: 'souvent forcenee et desmuee dentendement raisonnable et de tout sens'.

7 AN JJ 158 fo 11 no 20: 'laquelle elle aymoit tant que plus ne povoit quant elle estoit en bon sens'.

8 AN JJ 158 fo 11 no 20: 'navoit aucunne hayne aycelle ne aux amis delle'.

9 AN JJ 158 fo 11 no 20: 'quictons remectons et pardonnons ou cas dessusdit de notre grace especial et auctorite royal le fait et cas dessus dit avec toute peine offense et amende corporelle criminele et civile en quoy par rigueur elle pouvoit encourir evers nous et justice et la restituer a sa bonne fame et renommee au pais et a ses biens non confisquez en imposant sur ce silence perpetuel a notre procureur'.

Remission letters performed a particular legal function, by allowing stringent laws to be overturned in particular cases. Perhaps most significantly from the perspective of the supplicant, remission called for the reintegration of the criminal into his or her former position within society. The formula of the letters included a clause releasing the criminal from all corporal or civil punishment pertinent to the case. The crime was to be erased on the level of local justice, and it was to have no effect on the criminal's reputation. Clearly the crime could not be erased in reality. In cases of murder, like the one perpetrated by Jehannecte de la Forge, the victim would still be dead, and in cases of theft, even if stolen goods were returned, the crime would remain in the memories of the neighbors of the criminal. A royal decree could not truly affect communal memory, and the process of erasure included the public narration of the act that was supposed to be forgotten. Nevertheless, this legal erasure allowed people to return to their communities, either released from prison or returned from self-imposed exile. Indeed, the fact that remission was sought by individuals who had chosen to go into exile to escape from their crimes suggests the importance of the bonds of family and community. These supplicants implied in their letters that self-imposed exile was as much of a punishment as official banishment by the system of justice would have been.

Muriel Laharie, in her book on madness in the eleventh through thirteenth centuries, notes that the law allowed mad people to be released from prison if they recovered. She suggests, however, that most families would have preferred to leave their mad relatives in prison, paying for their upkeep, but otherwise free of the burden of caring for them, particularly since a recovery was no guarantee that the madness would not resurface later.[10] But the evidence from remission letters of the fourteenth and fifteenth centuries shows that many families preferred to have their relatives released into their care. Indeed, in most cases the mad people were still suffering from their illness when the family asked for them to be released from prison.

Fama

The choice to seek remission for a mad family member was not necessarily based entirely on sympathy or a desire to protect the mad person. Gaining remission involved a large investment of money and travel by the family. In addition, the family of the mad, in asking for the release of a mad person without punishment, was agreeing to take responsibility for controlling

10 Laharie 1991, pp. 253–255.

him or her in the future. In thinking about the motivations for the family to seek remission for their mad relatives, it is important to remember that in most remission letters, the criminal's feelings of shame came, not from having committed the criminal act, but from having been apprehended and imprisoned.[11] The shame of having a family member in prison or executed may have been more damaging to the reputation than caring for a mad relative in the household. Once a criminal case was brought to the attention of the local administrators of justice, the suspected perpetrator would be arrested and put in prison to await his or her trial. Often suspects would flee, essentially initiating a self-imposed exile since a decision to leave was taken as irrefutable proof of guilt. The concept of imprisonment as punishment was developing in this period, and it was occasionally cited as an alternative penalty if the culprit was incapable of paying the allotted fine.[12] Letters of remission reveal a strong fear of prisons and a recognition of time spent in prison as punishing, even if it was not officially used for that purpose in the context of the letter. Trials could be lengthy, and only the noble or wealthy could buy special treatment in prisons,[13] so some remission letters, highlighting the unpleasant conditions there, implied that punishment had already been meted out through a particularly long imprisonment. Remission letters often indicated further that the individual was likely to die before the completion of the trial, suggesting that prison could be a de facto capital punishment.

Remission rhetorically erased the crime, not only on the level of government officials, who could no longer pursue the pardoned criminal for that crime, but also on the level of the community, since the letter restored the criminal to his or her 'good reputation and renown'. The wider community's knowledge of an individual's character, as represented in common reputation and renown, was generally referred to in Latin sources as *fama* and in French as *fame* and *renomee*. *Fama*, or 'reputation', was a legal category that could affect a person and his or her family's standing in civil cases, ability to make contracts, and likelihood of conviction in criminal cases.[14]

11 Texier 2001, p. 485.

12 Dunbabin 2002, pp. 112–113. Dunbabin traces the development of the punitive function of prisons to the later twelfth and thirteenth centuries. Prisons were still mainly intended to confine people awaiting trial, however. See also Dean 2001, pp. 120–124.

13 Dunbabin 2002, p. 125. She notes, however, that the 'drawback to affluence' was that, regardless of the results of a trial, the wealthy were often forced to pay higher charges for release.

14 For an exploration of the development of the legal concept of *infama*, see Peters 1990. For an analysis focused more directly on France, particularly on the question of reputation in French customals, see Akehurst 2003. Daniel Smail has shown how reputation played a large role in both civil and criminal legal cases in Marseille, looking particularly at the ways in which witnesses' reputations could be challenged in order to erase their testimony, Smail 2003.

At the same time, 'reputation' was also a social category, determined by and affecting one's standing in the community.[15] Threats to an individual's reputation could threaten the reputation of the entire family, so the decision to seek remission for a mad family member may have been driven by a perceived need to restore the family's good standing in the community. Recent scholarship has revealed the multiple ways that an individual's *fama* or reputation could affect the prosecution and outcome of legal cases, both civil and criminal. According to Roman law, one of the ways to incur *infama* in its legal sense was by being convicted of a crime.[16] Indeed, bad *fama* could be a self-fulfilling prophesy, with those considered infamous in their community moving further and further into criminal activities, as David Chambers and Trevor Dean note in their discussion of criminality in fifteenth-century Italy.[17] The maintenance of good reputation was essential in an economy based on face to face interactions.

In theory, social reputation translated into legal reputation, since reputation and renown were proved in court through the use of witnesses who would testify to their own knowledge of the person. Thomas Kuehn argues, however, that 'there was no simple, direct, or automatic connection' between the two.[18] Rather, public reputation and common knowledge combined with the judges' knowledge of legal theories and discourse to create a legal category that was related to but not solely derived from communal consensus. Kuehn notes that the professional jurists and judges often determined what forms of common knowledge and reputation could 'count' in a legal setting: 'On the one hand, courts and jurists treated reputation and gossip as nonprofessional and resisted or limited their scope accordingly. On the other, common talk, properly disciplined, was one basis of proof and status.'[19] At a time when basic 'facts' of identity, such as birth dates, marriages, diseases (including madness), and deaths, were not necessarily recorded in written documents, witnesses' testimony about common knowledge was used to establish this information when it was pertinent to a case. Philippe de Beamanoir's book of customary law provides evidence that people's reputations (common knowledge of facts (*notoire*) and witness testimony to confirm these things) were central to legal practice.[20]

15 Hanawalt 1998, pp. 1–14.
16 Peters 1990, pp. 43–89; G.R. Evans 2002, pp. 123–129.
17 Chambers and Dean 1997, pp. 23–24.
18 Kuehn 2003, p. 27.
19 Kuehn 2003, p. 29.
20 Akehurst 2003.

Policing existed on a very basic level by this period, and particularly noticeable crimes were brought to the attention of the courts through a number of different avenues, only one of which was private denunciation. Laura Stern has shown that criminal cases in Florence were more likely to be initiated due to public *fama* (reputation), denunciation by an official, or inquisition *ex officio*, than by private accusation. Public reputation was not only the cause of the highest percentage of cases but also had the highest rate of conviction.[21] While the numbers certainly differ from place to place and from legal system to legal system, these percentages are suggestive of a larger pattern of accusation and conviction where *fama* was important for determining the outcome of trials. Communal knowledge was used to establish the details of a case, not just the reputation of the accused. During a court case, witnesses would be called to explain not only what they knew themselves but also what they considered 'common knowledge' in the community.

Professional jurists were not the only ones in a position to manipulate these categories, then. Witnesses could also control what they considered important 'common knowledge' in an effort to affect the outcome of legal cases, as Daniel Smail has demonstrated. Using civil cases in late medieval Marseille, he examines the ways that witnesses established the bad *fama* of the adverse party, and argues that the manipulation of reputations may even have been the ultimate goal of the litigant, which might explain the parties' willingness to undertake expensive and lengthy litigations. Sometimes the trials were not resolved at all, and even when they were the litigants often won less money than they had spent on the case.[22] However, the airing of differences in a public forum allowed the litigants to affect public knowledge and reputation through the legal case. The relationship between social *fama* and legal *fama* was circular, then, as each could affect the other.

The legal system both reflected and constructed communal rights and responsibilities. Community members depended upon one another for survival, but were also constantly competing over resources.[23] Ideals of neighborliness were a necessary part of life, and were policed as such. If people in the community agreed someone was of bad reputation their opinion could be sufficient for conviction in criminal cases, whereas good reputation could lead to acquittal, conviction for a lesser offense, or

21 Stern 1994, pp. 203–205.

22 Smail 2003, pp. 150–152.

23 David Sabean 1984 demonstrates this constant negotiation between neighborliness and conflict in early modern Germany.

conviction but with a lighter punishment. 'Common knowledge' had a role to play in jurisdiction. Almost all remission letters were constructed around the idea that the crime committed was not part of a criminal lifestyle. While the victims were sometimes described as individuals with bad reputations (*mala fama*), the perpetrators seeking remission were almost universally described as people of good reputation, who had never been accused or convicted of any previous crime. As a result, every letter to some degree describes and seeks to explain a moment of rupture. However, for those individuals identified as mad, the rupture was more extreme, and thus the explanation was even more exculpatory.

French customary law considered mad people potentially threatening to themselves and others. They recommended that the mad be guarded by their families and even by the community at large. Unlike Foucault's image of the wandering, isolated mad,[24] the law codes created an image of the mad as a central focus of communal concern.[25] The need to protect both the mad person and the community at large from the prospective damaging effects of madness underlay the recommendation that 'everyone' join together in a communal effort to guard the mad.[26] Mad people were considered communal burdens. Much like the customary law books, remission letters were written within the context of an 'imagined community' on the scale of the neighborhood and of the realm. These remission letters constructed images of communal involvement with madness. Neighbors' awareness of each other's lives invaded the home to consider the *gouvernance* of each member of the community. One of the explanations remission letters provided for why people who had been recognized as mad were able to commit crimes was because of *mal gouvernance*: the failure of their immediate family to care for them sufficiently. *Mal gouvernance* carried a wealth of censure in its connotations. It was used to describe women and men who did not care for their own children or who carried on adulterous affairs.[27] It also indicated a criminal negligence on the part of the household that would allow a man or woman who was only slightly wounded to die of those wounds.[28]

24 Foucault 2006, p. 9.

25 Rapetti 1850, p. 73, XXI.5.

26 Philippe de Beaumanoir 1970–1974, vol. 2, chapter 52, paragraph 1575; Gruchy 1881, p. 184, LXXIX.

27 See AN JJ 99 fo 33 no 104 (in 1367); AN JJ 176 fo 246 no 329 (in 1443); AN JJ 181 fo 55 no 100 (in 1452); AN JJ 204 fo 6v no 13 (in 1473).

28 See AN JJ 181 fo 19 no 34 (in 1451); AN JJ 181 fo 67v no 123 (in 1452); AN JJ 182 fo 18v no 33 (in 1453); AN JJ 182 fo 51v no 86 (in 1453).

A number of studies have established the significance of the household in the Middle Ages.[29] Households have been described as the basic economic unit of the Middle Ages, involving all members in the farming, craft, or trade of the whole.[30] Each member of the household, which was composed not only of a nuclear family but also included a variety of other members, such as extended family, servants, and apprentices, played a role in the smooth and efficient running of the business. These households were linked to each other through kinship, guilds, parishes, location in a town or city, and jurisdiction. Since, as David Herlihy has argued, society was ultimately made up of households,[31] the larger communities expressed concern about and attempted to impose controls on the households. Social interactions were based on *fama*, the rumored information that became common knowledge, regardless of factual truth, about each person and, often, spread to include his or her household. Composers of remission letters sought to establish the community's shared knowledge of the person who had committed a crime. In most cases, the reputation of the individual was established to be 'good'. However, in remission letters for mad criminals, often their mental state was confirmed by reference to common renown. This communal memory was sometimes evoked by reference to communal awareness of, concern about, and protection for the mad person's victims, or, in some situations, the mad person him- or herself.

Remission

Remission letters themselves provide the strongest evidence of the reconstruction of kin and communal bonds around the disruptive figure of the mad. These letters, composed by the family on behalf of the mad person, carried within their narratives a resolution that sought to restore the equilibrium of the local community. Because remission letters had to be read aloud by a local judge, the reconciliation was a public one. Despite, or indeed perhaps because of, the admission of guilt embedded within these letters that echoed public confession of sin, remission claimed to exonerate the criminal in the eyes of the community as a whole.

Jacques Mignon's remission letter, composed in 1458, described an unusual case, with a high level of community involvement.[32] According to the letter,

29 Many of these have focused on Italy. See Herlihy and Klapisch-Zuber 1985; and Hughes 1975. For peasant families in England, see Hanawalt 1986.

30 Herlihy 1983.

31 Herlihy 1985.

32 This case is also discussed in Pfau 2010b.

Jacques Mignon was known to be 'perturbed and altered in his senses',[33] but was well-loved by his neighbors in the small town of Richardère, near Bressuire in Poitou, because he would bring them pleasure by making (or doing) cartwheels.[34] When his wife, who was described as 'completely stupid, of simple and very small comportment, in such a manner that she does not know how to govern herself any better than a small child',[35] stopped riding into town with him in 1457, the townspeople brought her disappearance to the attention of the local officials.[36] Jacques was taken into custody and questioned, at which point he freely confessed that he had killed her. Jacques explained that she had asked to be taken to see her parents. They had begun the journey one night, leaving their five children asleep. Halfway there, he claimed, he had stopped the cart next to a river with a watermill and thrown her in the water, where she drowned. He had returned home alone and gone to sleep.

Jacques Mignon's free confession, without the use of torture, was considered suspect by the officers of the law. Since they had no other proof in addition to the mad man's confession, which was not considered legally valid testimony,[37] the local authorities could not proceed. They could not find a body, despite sending enquiries to the watermill to see if one had been discovered, and no one brought a case against Jacques Mignon for the death of his wife. The authorities were faced with a serious quandary as they tried to reconcile a need to protect the community against the possibly violent actions of a mad man and the need to protect the mad man from his own inability to comprehend reality. The remission letter was presented as a way to avoid dealing with a difficult legal situation. Jacques Mignon remembered killing his wife, and was fully capable of narrating the murder

33 AN JJ 188 fo 10 no 15, edited in Guérin 1909, vol. 10, pp. 92–94: 'perturbé et alteré de son entendement'.

34 It is unclear to me how making wheels for a cart would give pleasure to the people, which is why I suggest that he may have performed for them. AN JJ 188 fo 10 no 15, edited in Guérin 1909, vol. 10, pp. 92–94: 'et estoit amé au païs pour ce qu'il ce mesloit et entremettoit de faire roues de charette, et en ce et autres choses faisoit plusieurs plaisirs aux gens du païs d'ilec environ'.

35 AN JJ 188 fo 10 no 15, edited in Guérin 1909, vol. 10, pp. 92–94: 'toute sote, de simple et très petit gouvernement, en telle manière qu'elle ne se savoit gouverner, non plus que ung petit enfant'. Irina Metzler interprets this as 'the case of an "idiot" murdered by her insane husband'. Metzler 2016, p. 163. I would argue the narrative is more complex than that, and that the language used does not sufficiently distinguish between the two in the way Metzler asserts.

36 For more on denunciation by public *fama,* see Stern 1994, pp. 203–205.

37 This concept appeared in Justinian's code, Behrends, Knütel, and Mommsen 1995, vol. 1, pp. 78–80, Inst. 2.10, and was also brought into French customary law. See Philippe de Beaumanoir 1970–1974, vol. 1, chapter 12, paragraph 411 and vol. 2, chapter 34, paragraph 1061. See also Pfau 2010b.

when questioned about it. In his case, the local officers doubted whether his wife was actually dead, despite his belief that he had killed her. Jacques Mignon's willingness to confess to murder, apparently unaware of the penalties involved in such a confession, made the officers, who already knew from local repute that he was mad, unwilling to prosecute him for the crime without any further proof that his wife was dead. In the end, as the remission letter attests, they chose to protect the mad man, and the community banded together to seek a royal pardon for their entertaining friend, despite their awareness that he might have killed his wife.[38]

II. Community Concern: Chains, Cures, Recoveries, and Relapses

French customary laws expressed concerns about the potential dangers posed by mad people in their communities and recommended a variety of ways to cope, both before and after a crime had been committed. The *Ancienne Coutume de Normandie* made provisions for mad people who seemed likely to commit crimes, noting that

> If anyone is in such a way mad [*forsené*], that it is feared that he from his madness [*forcenerie*] might trouble the country, either by fire or by another thing that is contrary to the common health, he must be tied, and guarded by those who have his things, so that he does not wrong anyone; and if he has nothing, all the neighbors must give counsel and aid to his [family], to moderate his madness [*forcenerie*].[39]

The Norman customal was concerned about people who were mad 'in such a way' that they were considered likely criminals. Mad people were clearly considered communal burdens, since they were threatening to the 'common health'. In addition to the common concern that mad people might kill themselves or others, the Norman customal adds the fear that mad people might commit arson. Fire was clearly a major concern in communities made

38 Jacques Mignon was not a fool employed by the nobility, but he does appear to fulfill a similar function for the town of Richardère.

39 Gruchy 1881, p. 184, LXXIX: 'De Forcenés [...]. Se aulcun est en telle manière forsené, que l'en le doye doubter que de sa forcenerie il ne trouble le pays, ou par feu ou par aulcune chose qui soit contraire au commun salut, il doibt estre lié, et gardé par ceulx qui ont ses choses, qu'il ne mesface à nulluy; et s'il n'a rien, tout le voesiné doibt mettre conseil et aide du sien, à refréner sa forcenerie'.

of flammable materials, since a blaze begun in one house could quickly spread to the entire neighborhood. Thus, the entire neighborhood was responsible for surveillance of the mad, to prevent potential disasters, not only on an individual level, but also for the community at large.

Norman custom also suggested the community was responsible for the upkeep of a mad person, noting that '[i]f anyone is out of his senses, and he kills or injures a man by his madness [*forsenerie*], he should be put in prison, and be sustained by his [goods]; or it should be procured for him from the common alms, if he does not have anything with which he can be sustained'.[40] In Normandy, then, the community was expected to pay for the care of imprisoned mad criminals through their almsgiving, which suggests a very complicated attitude towards the mad. Here they appear as objects of pity, appropriate receivers of alms alongside the poor and lepers, but without the type of reciprocal relationship that almsgiving usually implied, where the prayers of the receiver were exchanged for the temporal support of the giver.[41] Not only would mad people be incapable of filling the role of grateful bedesmen and women, but also the legal text specifically indicates that this money was to be used for the care of a mad person who had been imprisoned because he or she had killed or injured another person. Thus, the uncomprehending criminal, who was incapable of prayer and whose inability to function normally in the world had injured or killed another person, somehow remained a reasonable recipient of community alms. The Norman customary law created a sense of communal responsibility through the figure of the mad criminal.

Like the Norman customal, Philippe de Beaumanoir also suggested imprisonment of the mad in order to prevent them from committing a crime, recommending that guardians take preventative action in the case of a person who 'went mad', rather than waiting until a crime had been committed. He explained that

> Those who are insane [*forsené*] should be bound by those who must guard them and everyone must help do this to avoid the damages that might come from them, for they could quickly kill themselves and others. And if they are not bound and they commit, because of their mad senses [*fol sens*], a homicide or any other serious crime, they are not punished like

40 Gruchy 1881, p. 184: 'De Forcenés. Se aulcun est hors du sens, et il occist ou mehaine ung homme par sa forsenerie, il doit estre mis en prison, et estre soustenu du sien; ou l'en luy doibt pourveoir des communes omosnes, s'il n'a de quoy il puisse estre soustenu'.

41 See Rubin 1987 and Mollat 1986.

> others because they do not know what they are doing, and their heirs do not for this reason lose what the insane [*forsenés*] person had, unless they had them in their care and it was done due to their inattention [*mauvais garde*]. But in any case the insane people [*forsenés*] must be placed in such a prison that they can never leave it, and be maintained from their own property as long as they are out of their senses [*hors du sens*]. And if he returns to his senses, he should be released from prison, and his goods returned to him.[42]

The focus here is clearly on the need to protect both the mad person and the community at large. Beaumanoir expressed a fear that mad people might commit suicide or murder, and that keeping such people bound or locked up would protect them and their community from their actions. In his view, all those who were insane contained within them the potential for such disruptive action. Interestingly, although Beaumanoir recommended that mad people be maintained from their own property, he also noted that 'everyone' must help to guard them, suggesting the need for a communal effort, much like the Norman customal. In contrast, a mid-fifteenth century customal from Anjou and Maine insisted that the perpetual imprisonment of a mad person should be paid for by the mad person.[43]

The *Livres de jostice*, in a departure from the other customals, held the family directly responsible for their mad relatives, suggesting that those who should have been guarding the mad be punished for the mad person's crimes:

> And if it is so, in the moment when he did the deed, that his friend had him in guard, such that he should have guarded him, you must call those who should have guarded him at the time when he did the deed: and if you find that he had been so negligent that by his negligence was the deed done, the law says that he must be put in punishment. – Because the guard of a mad person [*forsenez*] is given to his friends, not only so

42 Philippe de Beaumanoir 1970–1974, vol. 2, ch. 52, paragraph 1575: 'Cil qui sont forsené doivent estre lié par ceus qui les doivent garder et chascuns doit aidier a ce fere pour eschiver les damages qui par aus pueent venir, car tost ociroient aus et autrui. Et s'il ne sont lié et il font par leur fol sens aucun homicide ou aucun autre vilain cas, il ne sont pas justicié en la maniere des autres pour ce qu'il ne sevent qu'il font, ne leur oir ne perdent pas pour ce ce [sic] que li forsenés avoit, se ainsi n'est qu'il l'eussent en garde et que par leur mauvese garde li mesfès fu fes. Mes toutes voies li forsenés doit estre mis en tele prison qu'il n'en isse jamès, et soit soutenus du sien tant comme il sera hors du sens. Et s'il revient bien en son sens, il doit estre delivrés de prison, et li siens rendus'.

43 Beautemps-Beaupré 1883, p. 268.

> that he cannot do anything bad to himself, but so that he does nothing bad to others.
> And if the mad person [*desvé*] does something that he should not, the culpability should by right fall on those who should have guarded him, because he did that deed because of bad guard.[44]

The author of the *Livres de jostice* was invested in finding a responsible party to be blamed and punished for the criminal act. This potential reassignation of guilt may have been a driving force for family members seeking remission, since they may have feared they would be called to court for their relative's crime.

Community fears about the potentially dangerous actions of the mad occasionally translated into action in remission narratives. According to the remission letter Guillaume le Racif sought for his wife, Jehanne, she had been 'for a long time and on many occasions lunatic, frenzied, and insensible in such a way that she did not know how to maintain herself'.[45] Her madness was not constant, however, and she was considered capable of taking care of herself and her family during periods of sanity. One day in early April 1379, Jehanne le Racif was reportedly alone in the house with her four young children, when she was 'surprised by her said sickness'.[46] She picked up the youngest child, who was a baby girl aged six months, whom Jehanne had been breastfeeding, and hit the child on the stomach and sides until the baby died. Her other three children ran out of the house and cried out in the streets until a good neighbor woman heard them. She entered the house and found Jehanne 'completely enraged and insensible and supposed that from the said sickness she might do the same thing to her other children'.[47] The neighbor, clearly aware of the general *fama* about Jehanne's illness, acted to protect the family of the mad woman by

44 Rapetti 1850, p. 73 XXI.5: 'Et s'il est ensi, en tel point où il fit le fet, que si ami l'eussent en garde, qu'il le deussent garder, tu dois apeler cels qui le devient garder en cel tens qu'il fist le fet: et se tu trueves qu'il aient esté si négligent que par lor négligence soit li forfez fet, droiz dit que l'en les doit metre en poine. -- Quar la garde est baillie de forsenez à lor amis, non pas solement por aus qu'il facent mal, mès qu'il ne facent mal à autres.
Et se li desvé font chose qu'il ne doivent, l'en doit par droit metre lor colpes sor cels qui les doivent garder, comme il face tel fet par mauvèse garde'.

45 AN JJ 114 fo 106v no 212: 'de long temps souvente fois lunatique frenaisionse et incensible en tele maniere que elle ne scet son gouvernement'.

46 AN JJ 114 fo 106v no 212: 'fu de la dicte maladie surprise'.

47 AN JJ 114 fo 106v no 212: 'toute enragie et insensible et suppos len que par sa dict maladie elle eust ainsi fait de ses autre enfans qui ny feust seurvenu pour le quel fait ainsi advenu par meschief de la dicte maladie la dit Jehanne est prisonnier'.

intervening in the household and causing Jehanne to be arrested. She was put into prison in Orléans, where, because of her sickness, she had no idea where she was and insisted she had done nothing wrong.

Community networks were created as much by exclusion as by inclusion. In some cases a community's lack of care and concern for outsiders was cited as a cause of madness. Gouyn Cluchat's letter of 1459, discussed in detail below, demonstrated the possibility of failure in seeking help outside your own community.[48] When his family moved to a neighboring town to escape the plague, they ran out of provisions before it was safe to return. He decided to go into a nearby city to beg for food, but despite all his efforts, no one in this new town was willing to help him care for his family. As strangers and outsiders, Gouyn Cluchat's family had no recognized right to receive aid from their new neighbors. Indeed, community aid only arrived once the crisis reached its peak, and even then it did not alleviate the original problem. Cluchat became suicidal, attempting to drown himself in a fountain in the town. A woman passing by stopped to ask him what he was doing, expressing concern, but too late to help Cluchat, who fled. Instead of killing himself, he returned home and, 'as if he was out of his senses', killed his wife with an axe.[49]

His neighbors did not offer support, and even after he killed his wife, they refused to act for or against him. Cluchat told them he had just killed his wife and asked them to have him arrested. Indeed, when they refused, he went even further, traveling to the nearby city of Combronde and demanding they put him to death for his crime. At this moment, when it was no longer possible to save Cluchat's wife, his extended family, who for reasons unmentioned in the letter had not been available to give him provisions, proffered aid by seeking remission on his behalf. Given the price of a remission letter, this generosity was too much too late. His letter, like many others, leaves us with no clear picture of his ultimate fate. He was released from prison on the authority of the king, and with no conditions such as keeping him chained up or under guard. His family seemed to believe his release would prevent his children from becoming beggars, but they provided no hint about what would be done to cope with his extreme depression and his desire to be punished for his crime. Cluchat's decision to leave his local network and seek aid elsewhere was the source of his difficulties.

Despite these difficulties in seeking communal aid outside one's home village, the narratives in the remission letters suggest that local neighborly

48 AN JJ 188 fo 81 no 160.

49 AN JJ 188 fo 81 no 160: 'come hors du sens et debilite de son entendement'.

aid was generally expected to be forthcoming. The responsibility of guarding mad people, particularly those who were suspected of suicidal tendencies, rested with the immediate household, but there is ample evidence that the assistance of neighbors was sought and, very often, provided. Generally this neighborly aid arose in the context of a tale about a failed attempt at preventing suicide, as the mad person escaped and died. Usually this guardian duty fell on the local women, perhaps as an extension of their work as nurses. Symonnette aux Beufs came to watch over the sickbed of Jehan Massetirer in 1394. Earlier in the day, Jehan had left the house and attempted to drown himself in the river, but he was saved by his wife and two men passing by. Left alone with Symonnette, Jehan got out of bed, completely naked (a detail that seems intended to reinforce his madness, since he was willing to walk around naked in front of a neighbor woman), and hit her over the head, knocking her down. He ran out of the house, jumped into a well nearby, and was drowned before anyone could pull him out.[50] Another case described a number of controls put in place by Robert Senuminem's wife and close family to prevent him from harming himself or others. In this case, the guards came from within the household. Robert, 'during his life by intervals and some times for a very long time was furious'.[51] As a result, his close family placed people in his household to 'keep him company so as to guard him'.[52] Nevertheless, after hearing the mass on Tuesday, 28 April 1404, his family explained that he returned home, convincing the chamber maid he wanted to sleep. When she left him in bed, he got up and hanged himself, despite the valiant attempts made to prevent him from achieving his aim.

Although setting guards over sickbeds was a common practice, the remission letters suggest that some family members were reluctant to go so far as to chain the mad before they exhibited extreme violent behavior. The need to keep mad people in chains was written into the customary laws of a number of regions of France. Indeed, a few remission letters mention chains provided by the local representative of justice or by the family for people who were known to be mad for a long period of time before their crime. Perrim de Moustier was given chains by the marshal of Pontoise to chain his son.[53] However, after Jehan de Moustier broke out of those chains, Perrim refused to continue to restrain him. Similarly, the remission letter for Jehannecte

50 AN JJ 146 fo 65 no 129.

51 AN JJ 158 fo 165 no 303: 'ou temps de sa vie par intervales et aucune fois de longs a longs este furoieux'.

52 AN JJ 158 fo 165 no 303: 'pour lui tenir compaigne afin de le garder'.

53 AN JJ 118 fo 18v no 18.

Troppé stated that her husband refused to chain her, hoping she would return to her 'bon sens' and life in their household would go back to normal. Both of these men were ultimately victims of violent, frenzied attacks by their son and wife, respectively, and the composers of the remission letters, with knowledge of the ultimate outcome, blamed the victim to some extent for refusing to ensure that the mad person could not become so violent.

Chaining the mad could backfire, however, especially since some cases of madness were seen as cyclical. Guille Crieusch's wife was out of her senses such that, he claimed, he feared she would do something bad. In 1411, he applied to the duke of Burgundy, who had jurisdiction over Guille's town of Houlle near Amiens, requesting and receiving a license to constrain his wife. He kept her locked up for six weeks, after which she appeared to return to her good senses, and even 'sometimes went to church and did her work as other women do'.[54] She seemed so well recovered, Guille explained, that he left her alone one evening with their children. After he left, she picked up an ax or 'another utensil with a sharp point'[55] and killed one of their children and chased the others, who cried loudly enough to bring the neighbors to the house. Interestingly, perhaps because Guille's wife was registered as mad and he was supposed to be responsible for preventing her from doing anything wrong, it was Guille who was brought before the justice to account for the crime, and was, he claimed, in danger of being banished for not taking sufficient care of his mad wife, forcing the neighbors to intervene to save his children.

The cyclical nature of some forms of madness made any sort of guard a difficult prospect. During their periods of sanity, mad people were allowed to return to their normal lives, and many remission letters established that the person had suffered from bouts of insanity, but was considered recovered, and therefore was unguarded, when the madness returned and the crime was committed. Cases of suicide described elaborate ruses the mad person set up to send everyone away from the house so he or she was no longer being guarded. Keeping the mad from harming themselves or others through restraints or surveillance was not easy, then, but seeking a cure could be even more difficult.

Attempts to cure madness most often involved visits to saints' shrines.[56] Often, the mad would be taken to several shrines when a cure was not

54 AN JJ 166 fo 64 no 100: 'aloit aucuneffoiz aleglise et faisoit sa besongne comme les autres femmes font'.

55 AN JJ 166 fo 64 no 100: 'autre ostil dun charpoint'.

56 In his study of miracle stories, Sigal 1985, pp. 236–239, conflates possession and madness, but notes that 91% of the cures took place in the presence of the saint or of the saint's relics.

forthcoming. Just as shrine records sometimes included stories of failed medical cures that were triumphed over by the successful spiritual cure,[57] remission letters tell us about ultimately unsuccessful pilgrimages. Although there were saints considered particularly good at curing madness, most of the pilgrimages recorded in remission letters were focused locally, at shrines close to home. This is unsurprising, particularly when one considers the potential difficulties of traveling with a mad person. Foucault's image of solitary mad people wandering the roads and waterways of Europe on their way to shrines is not supported by the evidence in these letters, which suggests rather that pilgrimages would be undertaken in groups of at least two, including one healthy individual, generally a member of the family. Indeed, as Irina Metzler notes in her study of disability in medieval Europe, many miracle seekers traveled with the aid of others.[58]

Several of the saints known for curing madness were French saints, so they were ideally located for more local pilgrimages. Saint Mathurin of Larchant's shrine is seventy-eight kilometers (forty-nine miles) south of Paris. Charles VI's queen, Isabeau de Bavière, stopped there in 1416 on a lengthier pilgrimage, possibly to pray for her husband's health.[59] One remission letter from 1422 described a pilgrimage to St. Mathurin undertaken by a mad man and his relatives.[60] Guille Cliquet lived in Talon-Judas near Saint-Pere-le-Moustier, about 157 kilometers (ninety-eight miles) from St. Mathurin de Larchant and 228 kilometers (142 miles) from Paris. In the letter written on his behalf, his relatives and close family explained that he

> had been furious and out of his senses for some time and for diverse intervals. Because of these things he was put in irons, chained, and taken to Saint Mathurin of Larchant and on other pilgrimages and sometimes he came to convalescence and afterwards he fell back into his lunacy. The which Cliquet, when he is in health, is a very good, diligent laborer and a man of great care.[61]

57 Ronald Finucane 1977, p. 59, found that one in ten pilgrims to shrines in England had sought medical aid previously. See also an interesting combination: the physician-saint Gil de Santarem in McCleery 2005.

58 Metzler 2006, pp. 169–176.

59 Verdier 1969, p. 33.

60 AN JJ 171 fo 292 no 520.

61 AN JJ 171 fo 292 no 520: 'ait este furieux et hors de son sens par aucuns temps et par divers intervalles pour ocasion desquel choses il aeste enferre lie et meue asaint mathurin de larchant et en autres pelerinages et aucuneffoiz en est venu a convalescence et depuis par lunoisons y est rancheu le quel cliquet quant il est en sante est un tresbon laboureur diligent et homme de grant peine'.

Guille Cliquet's illness was considered cyclical, and related to the phases of the moon. While his family tried to find a resolution to the problem by taking him on multiple pilgrimages, even the saints could only aid him for a time before he would again fall into madness.

However, despite the failure of holy remedies, Guille Cliquet was a diligent worker during his periods of sanity. The letter further revealed that Guille lived in a household with his brothers, who held their beasts in common, providing an environment in which Guille could work when he was able, and presumably supporting him, along with his wife and children, when he was not. Indeed, the crime that led his relatives to seek remission for him was intimately involved in the household arrangements. A group of soldiers came through town, appropriating the local beasts and destroying outbuildings.[62] While they were at Guille Cliquet's home, they tore down the household's stone well. According to the letter, Cliquet was at this time 'in his senses', but he was naturally very angry, and set about repairing the well the evening the soldiers left town, with his son holding a candle to provide light for the task. Fortunately, many of their cattle had been saved because their valet, Guille Talart, had taken them into the hills to hide, and he also returned to the household that night. As Cliquet's relatives described the scene in his letter of remission, Talart insisted on taking the light Cliquet was using, going so far as to wrest it from Cliquet's son's hands. Cliquet, who was already angered by the actions of the soldiers, entered into his fury and attacked Talart, giving him a wound from which he eventually died. The healing powers of the saint were not sufficient to prevent Cliquet from acting out of proportion to the situation.

Jehan de Moustier, whose story is detailed in Chapter Two, was also taken to a saint's shrine and was disruptive while there.[63] His father, Perrim, took him to the shrine of Saint Titenerd at Gournay, north of their home in Saint-Denis. At the saint's shrine, Jehan de Moustier was chained up and left to await God's mercy, but he escaped from those chains and ran away. When he was recaptured, his family returned him to the shrine where they applied two sets of chains, but even this was not enough to hold Jehan, who had strength enough to escape from those as well. Clearly, the saint was not able to provide a cure at this time, and Perrim de Moustier took him back home.

62 I discuss some aspects of this case in Pfau 2013b.

63 Finucane 1977, pp. 107–109, also describes the disruptive behavior of mad people at saint's shrines, which seems to have been a common theme in miracle records as well as in remission letters.

The *Chronicle of Saint Denis* described the successful cure of a disruptive madman at Saint Denis's shrine. It is worth contrasting the successful community healing ritual described by a monk with the unsuccessful rituals seen in remission letters. Again, the pilgrimage was a local one, so it was the man's neighbors who brought him to the shrine and witnessed the cure:

> [f]or a certain baker of the city of St. Denis had lost his inner sense, and captured by a demon, foaming and crying with a terrible voice, any who wanted to approach him or come to him, like an ungoverned savage beast, he tried to tear into morsels with great ferocity. So his relatives and neighbors led him, bound with iron chains, to the church of the holy martyr, and placed him before the image of the crucifix. They said prayers and his mad fury calmed a little. Then they guided him before the altar of the martyr, where for a little while he lay down on the ground, as if separated from his bodily senses. Suddenly from his mouth a fetid breath exited, and then getting up with hilarity, on bended knees, he gave thanks to God and to the glorious martyr, affirming publicly to all that he through invocation of the saint recovered his whole health.[64]

His family and neighbors brought him to the shrine in hopes of recovery, perhaps especially because the baker held an important economic position within the local community. The image of communal involvement the chronicler paints here is compelling. These 'family and neighbors' were actively involved in helping him to get to the shrine, binding him and dragging him along with them. Together, the mad man and the saint helped to initiate and confirm communal unity.

Just because other people aided in the pilgrimage does not mean that everyone was supportive, caring, and understanding of mad pilgrims. Indeed, just as remission letters reveal failed pilgrimages, they also uncover

64 Bellaguet 1842, vol. 1, pp. 314–316: 'Quidam namque panificus de villa beati Dyonisii sensum penitus amiserat, et arreptus a demone, spumans ac terribilibus vocibus clamans, volentes ad ipsum accedere vel eidem occurrentes, velud effrenis belua, ferocissimis morsibus conabatur discindere. Quem cum cathena ferrea ligatum amici et vicini ad ecclesiam beati martiris attulissent, coram ymagine crucifixi, oracionibus factis, aliquantulum vesanum impetum deposuit. Deinde eum ante altare martiris perducentes, cum super pavimentum aliquandiu jacuisset, velud a corporeis sensibus segregatus, subito ex ore ejus anhelitus fetidissimus exivit, et tunc hylariter surgens, flexis genibus, gracias Deo egit et glorioso martiri, publice cunctis affirmans quod ejus precibus receperat integram sanitatem'.

failed attempts at cementing civic unity. One case in particular provides evidence that not all miracle seekers were fortunate enough to have a considerate network of family and neighbors. Instead, a stranger verbally and physically abused Margot, who was suffering from the malady of Saint John, often called Saint John's Dance.[65] According to a letter written in 1379 on behalf of Jehan Dargilles, a bystander who came to her defense, Margot arrived at the church of Saint John the Baptist in Sens on the saint's feast day (24 June) with a group of others suffering from the dancing sickness. Standing in front of the shrine of Saint John, Margot 'burdened and much aggrieved by the said illness, took the candles placed before the image of the said Saint John and broke them, destroyed them, and threw them to the ground like an insensible person without reason'.[66] Another resident of Sens, Huguenin Vice Serviter, took offense at Margot's actions and verbally abused her, saying that if he met her outside the church he would hit her. Jehan Dargilles 'moved by pity for the said Margot, for consideration and compassion of her said illness, strongly blamed the said Serviter for the words and threats that he had said and made to the said Margot'.[67] Although the two men left the church peaceably enough, they met later in the street and began a brawl that led to Huguenin Vice Serviter's death at Jehan Dargilles' hands.

In their attempts to cure the mad the community preferred religious to medical aid. Though madness was certainly seen as a malady, and even described in humoral terms, remission letters rarely mention active medical intervention. Only one letter out of the 155 examined mentioned medicine as instrumental in curing a mad person, and even in this case the reference is ambiguous. In his madness, Robert Layne would go out into the woods

65 There were several outbreaks of the dancing sickness in the Middle Ages and into the early modern period. E. Louis Backman 1977, pp. 170–258, discusses them all in detail. On pages 190–216 he discusses an epidemic in 1374 in Flanders, Germany, and France, and argues on pages 303–327 that the dancers in all these epidemics actually suffered from ergot poisoning. He does not mention any outbreaks in 1379, and in fact tends to argue that any chronicles providing alternative dates to the dates of the larger outbreaks were mistaken, perhaps in order to strengthen his argument about ergotism. Erik Midelfort 1999, pp. 32–49, also discusses Saint Vitus's Dance, which is a later incarnation of the dancing sickness (the name St. Vitus's Dance does not appear until the sixteenth century).

66 AN JJ 115 fo 73 no 154: 'chargee et mout agreuse du dit mal prenent les chandelle mises devant lymage du dit saint jehan et les cussart desrompoit et gectoit aterre comme personne insensee et sans raison'.

67 AN JJ 115 fo 73 no 154: 'meu de pitie envers la dite margot pour consideracion et compassion de sa dite maladie blasma fortement le dit serviter de parolles et menaces quil avoit dites et faites ala dite margot'.

naked with rocks in his hands and threaten to kill anyone who came near him, so that

> no one dared to approach him except the Seigneur and Dame de Campergny who thus brought him to live in their hostel. He took him or had him taken and tied him or had him tied such that by medicine or otherwise in the custody of God he came back to himself and had cognizance.[68]

Once he was brought home, he decided to go on a pilgrimage to Saint Acorée. In the end, however, neither the medical nor the religious cure was sufficient, since, according to his remission letter from 1387, any time he was angered he would become uncontrollable and frenetic. Physicians were never called in as experts to provide proof of madness, although they were called as witnesses for other physical illnesses,[69] and in the fourteenth century physicians were brought into the court to provide testimony in the form of prognosis for the injured party, determining whether or not the wounds were likely to prove fatal.[70]

Family care was clearly considered a better option than prison, where (at least according to the rhetoric of the remission letters) the prisoner was likely to die, whether or not he or she was ultimately convicted. Although care within the household could involve chains and cells, it could also involve pilgrimages or treatments to seek a cure that would have been unavailable in prison. In addition, a mad person who recovered could be returned to his or her previous position. Because medieval people believed madness was a disease from which people could and did recover, and because most of these remission letters were written for people who had contributed to the support of their immediate families before they became mad, it is likely they were closely observed in the hopes they would recover.

However, even if caring for the mad within the household was preferable, it was certainly not without its own pitfalls. Indeed, sometimes the stress of caring for the mad was enough to bring a household to a point of crisis. Jacquet Morniet's sister-in-law became so annoyed about having to care for him while he was bed-ridden with melancholy in 1459 that she made the

68 AN JJ 131 fo 103 no 166. Edited in Saunier 1993, p. 498: 'par ce nul ne l'osoit aprouchier se ne fust le Seigneur et Dame de Campergny qui ainsi comme il se vint bouter en leur hostel ilz le poindrent ou firent prendre et le lièrent ou firent lier tant que par médicine ou aultrement que à la garde de Dieu il se revint et ot cognoissance'.

69 AN JJ 171 no 411. Edited in Longnon 1878, p. 17. Note that Longnon does not provide folio references.

70 Tanon 1877, pp. 18–19.

mistake of berating him, calling him worthless and lazy.[71] Enraged, Jacquet hit her with a stick and killed her. This remission letter is an excellent example of the optimism of the composers of remission letters. Jacquet's family asked for his release so he could help care for his wife and children. Yet before his crime, he was unable to support himself and was relying on his brother's charity. This fraternal care would presumably not be forthcoming after his release, however, since his brother was instrumental in his arrest. Jacquet's family must have been hoping (or expecting) he would recover from his illness and become a useful member of the community once more, despite the unpleasant results of his dependence on his brother.

This negative response of household members to caring for the mad was not unusual. A letter composed in 1482 on behalf of Regnaulde des Vieulx, twenty-four or twenty-five year-old widow of Pierre Pelletier, explained that she had been living in the household of her husband's parents after his death. In addition to Regnaulde and her child, the household included her father-in-law, his daughter, Begnoiste, and her husband, Odile Deleslang. Begnoiste, who was only fourteen years old, was described in the letter as 'foolish and insensible, and not pleasing to the said Odile',[72] who was more interested in the older widow. Odile and Regnaulde began to have an affair, and Odile suggested that he should kill Begnoiste so they could marry. In the remission letter written on her behalf, Regnaulde claimed to have protested against this plan, but agreed that if by chance Begnoiste were to die, she would be happy to be Odile's wife. When Begnoiste was discovered drowned in a nearby fountain, Odile left town, thereby confirming his culpability, since the choice of voluntary exile was equivalent to an admission of guilt. When the officers of Neuilly came to question Regnaulde, the private lives of the Pelletier household became public knowledge.

The remission letters narrated the discomforts of dealing with mad people, along with the attempts made to help them. These awkward figures threatened their communal and kinship ties, but at the same time they could be used as symbols of and cement for those same bonds. Mad people were expected to recover and reaffirm their identities as integral parts of the larger community. The attempts made to hasten that recovery through pilgrimage or to guard the mad to prevent them from harming themselves or others placed the mad person at the center of communal concern. This communal concern was perhaps most clear in a particular type of crime narrative that began to appear in the middle of the fifteenth century, in

71 AN JJ 188 fo 102 no 203.

72 AN JJ 209 fo 61 no 104: 'folle et incensee et nestoit pas ala plaisance dudit odile'.

which the mad person became an impetus for vigilante justice, not as its victim, but as its cause.

III. Acts of Communal Justice: Sorcerers and Remission

Towards the middle of the fifteenth century, a new narrative phenomenon began to appear in the remission letters. These letters were written on behalf of individuals and, often, large groups of people guilty of murder, who insisted that their victims were 'renowned' sorcerers.[73] These accusations of sorcery and bewitchment, nonexistent in the earlier letters, included references to proofs of the sorcerer's power in the community, describing cases of impotence, infertility, and madness.[74] The supplicants generally sought remission for what they presented as a cooperative effort to interrogate the accused sorcerer, leading to the sorcerer's death from exposure or other 'natural' causes.

The descriptions of behavior of those driven mad through sorcery could be distinctively different from that of those whose madness was attributed to other causes. Some victims of sorcery are depicted unthreateningly, as 'madly running naked through the fields',[75] and one letter connected the bewitched man's impotence to his madness,[76] but often the letters voiced a fear that this madness caused by bewitchment would lead the victim to take his or her own life.[77] These letters had a very different focus from those composed for mad criminals. Although there are a few exceptions where the mad person lashed out at the accused sorcerer, most letters seek forgiveness for family members who sought to remove the bewitchment through actions that 'accidentally' resulted in the accused sorcerer's death. Therefore, the mad were incidental to the crime, and these bewitched mad people appeared as much more sympathetic figures than the mad who committed crimes themselves. These narratives inverted the typical themes of madness, where a family member was the victim of a criminal attack by the mad, into a story of the family member as the active participant in an act of violence focused outside the family circle on a 'renowned' sorcerer.

73 I have written more on the subject of attacks on sorcerers in Pfau 2013a.

74 For more on the connection between impotence, magic, and witchcraft, see Rider 2006, pp. 186–207.

75 AN JJ 187 fo 89v no 173 (in 1457): 'courroit folle parmy les champs toute nue'.

76 AN JJ 208 fo 11 no 20 (in 1480).

77 See AN JJ 199 fo 276 no 441 (in 1464); AN JJ 227 fo 32 no 62 (in 1496).

In a letter composed in 1496, Petit Jehan Secretani described the events that led him to kill Estienne Mollet.[78] Petit Jehan's sister, Jehanne, had married three years before and immediately 'fallen into a great misfortune of sickness such that she was strongly troubled in her sense and understanding and was completely senseless and in danger each day of harming herself and the fruit with which at that time she was pregnant'.[79] According to the letter, this illness meant her family could have no joy together. Petit Jehan saw the source of her madness outside the immediate family, but nevertheless linked to her through fellowship. Estienne Mollet, known by the community as a sorcerer able to cure a number of diseases, was often in the company of their father, Estienne Secretani, and with access to Jehanne's food, which Petit Jehan Secretani believed he had poisoned. The simultaneous rupturing and cementing of familial and community ties were stressed throughout this letter, as Petit Jehan joined Jehanne's brother-in-law, Laurens Grenault, in beating up Estienne Mollet while demanding he give them information about the bewitchment of their sister.

Studies of witchcraft accusations in diverse locations have noted that, while the educated inquisitors and judges were most concerned with the question of worship of the devil, most accusers were focused on the details of the evil deeds performed through magic.[80] The social aspects of magical acts, rather than a theological insistence on heretical beliefs, were important to those who brought cases against their neighbors. While the dangers of heresy in the community were certainly clear to the inquisitors, since heretics were believed to seek converts and could thus corrupt their neighbors, the dangers of sorcery were obvious to all, since they actively worked to attack their neighbors. Norman Cohn argues that the lack of witchcraft accusations in the Middle Ages was due not to a lack of belief in popular culture, but rather to the legal system of 'talion', whereby the accuser, if unable to convince the judge of the guilt of the accused, would suffer as heavy a penalty as fit the crime. He cites the evidence of lynchings from the ninth century into the eleventh to prove there was a widespread belief in witchcraft before the

78 AN JJ 227 fo 32 no 62 (in 1496).

79 AN JJ 227 fo 32 no 62: 'cheult en grant inconvenant de maladie tellement quelle fut fort troublee de son sens et entendement et estoit toute incensee et en dangier de chacun jour precipiter elle et le fruit dont pour lors estoit ensaincte'.

80 Edward Peters 2002, p. 218, notes for the fourteenth century: 'In secular courts generally, jurists looked for damage actually caused by sorcery; in ecclesiastical courts canonists looked for indications that sorcery was practised by means that clearly savoured of heresy, especially the homage paid to demons in return for magical powers'. See also Briggs 1989; Briggs 1996; Cohn 1975; Karlsen 1987.

trials.[81] Significantly, however, the fifteenth-century French remission letters about the killing of sorcerers (or the accidental death of people rumored to be sorcerers) appear in the archive even after witchcraft trials had already begun in parts of Switzerland and eastern France.[82]

The devil had a strong presence in letters of remission at least from Charles V's reign, which marks the beginning of this study. The 'temptation of the enemy' did not excuse an action, but it did provide a reasonable motivational force for the crime. Natalie Zemon Davis, in her study of later remission letters, notes that the phrase was no longer in use in the sixteenth century.[83] The coincidence of an increasing interest in the connection of the devil with sorcery and witchcraft in this period suggests that the 'temptation of the enemy' may have become a more troubling claim in the sixteenth century than in the fifteenth. It was still occasionally used in oral depositions at trials, but the more composed format of the remission letters perhaps edited out such references.

Jean Gerson and other fourteenth-century theologians interested in the discernment of spirits believed that possession, whether by God or by the devil, manifested itself in behavior very similar to madness.[84] The concern of these theologians was to determine which of the three possibilities was in fact occurring in a particular case and to act accordingly, whether to beatify, exorcise, or call a physician.[85] Fifteenth-century scholars shifted attention to the capabilities of sorcerers, rather than the direct actions of the devil.

81 Cohn 1975, pp. 160–163.

82 Paravy 1979. Bernard Gui's inquisitorial manual in the early fourteenth century mentions witchcraft, but he never convicted any witches. See Cohn 1975, p. 131. Nicolas Eymerich wrote his *Directorium Inquisitorum* in 1376. His manual for inquisitors discussed witchcraft, but only as one among many heresies. His focus was on the distinction between *dulie* and *latrie* of the devil, or worship (which is due only to God) and veneration (which is applicable to the saints). These two different levels of heretical behavior in the practice of sorcery determined the appropriate punishment for the sorcerer. Jean Gerson's treatise written in 1402, *De erroribus circa artem magicam*, circulated with the appended articles condemning magic by the University of Paris in 1398.

83 Davis 1987, p. 37. See also the corresponding endnote number 6 on pages 169–170.

84 Gerson 1962, vol. 3, p. 39.

85 Most modern work on this topic has been more interested in the first two possibilities. See Caciola 2003; Caciola 2000; Newman 1998. However, madness was also a viable diagnosis. Friar Felix Fabri wrote of a visit to a small town in Germany: 'In the village of Jedensheim, or Iheidemsheim, at the foot of the hill on which the castle stands, there was a maiden bereft of her reason, whom many declared to be possessed of a devil; he showed me this maiden for me to look at and examine, that I might decide what was to be done with her; whether she ought to be exorcised or not. My decision was that she was out of her mind, and therefore fitter to be entrusted to the care of physicians than to that of theologians'. Fabri 1896, vol. 1, p. 56.

Sorcerers were believed capable not only of channeling demonic possession, but also of causing physical illnesses, including madness, through potions and spells. Johan Nider wrote his *Formicarius* sometime around 1437. In this treatise, he explained miraculous and marvelous events, introduced with brief allegorical interpretations of the behavior of ants.[86] In Book Five, Chapter Three, the Theologian presented to his interrogator, the Lazy One, the kinds of damages sorcerers can inflict through their demons. He explained:

> [t]hen, the first manner works to create in a man an illicit love for a woman or in the contrary sense, in a woman for a man. Another serves to provoke hatred or jealousy in someone. The third is found in those who are called ensorcelled, because the men and women cannot use their generative force. The fourth manner is to make a man suffer in one of his members. The fifth deprives him of his life. The sixth deprives him of the use of his reason. The seventh is to harm him by attacking his goods or his animals.[87]

This list of harmful acts reflects an intense concern about reproduction, relationships, and household resources, as well as a fear of attacks on the individual. Unlike the general run of heretics, sorcerers were visibly damaging to the community, regardless of whether they were actively recruiting. Nider listed deeply threatening powers over people's relationships with others, since sorcerers could control love, hatred, or jealousy, all of which could be instilled in another person without cause or reference to the ordinary balance of the community. Equally, an inability to reproduce threatened the continuity of a household, and through that household of the community as a whole, just as the destruction of property and household resources did.

Similarly, loss of reason was a serious threat to the cohesiveness of the community, since mad people were perceived as likely to attack ties of

86 Chène 1999, p. 106. The titles of the five books are *Libellus primus principaliter erit de raris bonorum hominum exemplis et operacionibus, Secundus de verisimilibus bonis revelacionibus, Tercius de falsis et illusoriis visionibus, Quartus de virtuosis perfectorum operacionibus, Quintus de maleficis et eorum decepcionibus.*

87 Nider 1999, pp. 148–149: 'Unus igitur modus est quo amorem malum ingerunt viro alicui ad mulierem aliquam, vel mulieri ad virum. Alius est cum odium vel invidiam in aliquo seminare procurant. Tercius est in his qui maleficiati dicintur, ne vi generativa uti valeant ad feminam vel viceversa femelle ad virum. Quartus est cum in membro aliquo hominem egrotare faciunt. Quintus cum vita privant. Sextus quando usu racionis aliquem privant. Septimus cum quocumque predictorum modorum aliquem in suis rebus vel animalibus'.

community and kinship, thus furthering the larger goal of the sorcerer. In the end, attacking an individual's life or body parts seems the least disruptive possibility.

It may be theologically significant that Nider chose to say sorcerers could deprive a person of the 'use of his reason', not actually deprive him of his reason. Although the sorcerer was able to create an impediment to using reason, they were not able to actively threaten a person's reason. Indeed, Nider provided an exemplum about the judge Pierre in Berne, who was injured by means of sorcery. Pierre was generally quite careful about protecting himself with his faith and constant signing of the cross, but one night he woke up in the middle of the night and left himself open to the devil. Believing it was morning due to some 'fictive light', he went downstairs and found the front door locked. Angered at his attendants, he returned up the stairs cursing, saying 'In the name of the devil'. Immediately, Pierre fell back down the stairs onto his head. He was found 'deprived of the use of his reason, wounded everywhere and bleeding profusely'.[88] This story was used by Nider to demonstrate that even holy men, despite their best efforts, can slip up occasionally, allowing sorcerers and the devil access to them. However, perhaps the most interesting aspect is that Pierre's wounds and loss of reason were by-products of the sorcerer's act, which was to make him trip on the stairs. Although sorcerers had the power to wound people remotely, they were also capable of taking advantage of dangerous situations. Pierre eventually regained the use of his reason through God's grace, and recovered from his other wounds.

Heinrich Institoris, who wrote the *Malleus Maleficarum* in 1484, was heavily influenced by Nider's work.[89] He also explained that witches were capable of inflicting illness on their victims. Institoris, however, was particularly intent on proving that witches could cause epilepsy and leprosy, because, as he pointed out, physicians claimed these diseases generally arose from longstanding preconditions, and therefore were unlikely to be contracted through supernatural means.[90] Interestingly, in his discussion of how sorcerers could cause illnesses, he devoted relatively little space to madness, merely stating '[t]he situation with harming the use of reason and harassing the internal senses is made clear through the case of the

88 Nider 1999, pp. 190–193: 'luce deceptus ficticia'; 'In nomine dyaboli'; 'privatum racionis usu iacentem et collisum per omnia membra, sanguinem plurimum e corpore emittentem'.

89 For more on the *Malleus* and its wider influence, see Broedel 2003. There is a scholarly debate on whether Jacobus Sprenger coauthored the *Malleus*. See Maxwell-Stuart 2007, pp. 30–31.

90 Institoris and Sprenger 2006, vol. 2, p. 311.

possessed and "stricken," as well as by Gospel stories'.[91] Thus, sorcery could cause madness, since it was clear the devil could cause cases of possession by targeting a person's 'use of reason'.

The narratives in letters of remission about witchcraft revolved around issues of trust, threat, and reputation in the community. They revealed and simultaneously sought to mend deep fissures in the ideals of communal support. The mad person, along with other perceived victims of malefaction, became the central figures of a narrative of communal reconstruction at the expense of the reputed sorcerer. However, the letters also illuminate the roles that sorcerers were expected and even, occasionally, required to play in the neighborhood. Generally, these sorcerers were sought out originally on the pretext of desiring magical healing, not because they were immediately presumed to be the cause of the illness. It was only after the sorcerer's attempts failed, or he or she[92] refused to help, that the narratives escalated into violence.[93] Like the mad person in narratives of mad crime, the sorcerer had a role to play that was acceptable in certain prescribed ways.

In 1464, Jehan Sommet, a notary living in the town of Thiart in Auvergne, sought remission for the crime of murder. He described his troubling night on the twelfth or thirteenth of June, when his wife 'was greatly troubled in her sense and understanding, crying with a loud voice as if insensible, and wishing to throw herself out the windows into the street'.[94] Jehan Sommet explained that he called his neighbors to aid him in guarding his wife and preventing her from doing herself harm. He claimed he made a number of vows, to both male and female saints, on his wife's behalf, but they did not

91 Institoris and Sprenger 2006, vol. 2, p. 307; The Latin is from Institoris and Sprenger, vol. 1, p. 457: 'Item de nocumento vsus rationis et vexatione interiorum sensuum probatur ex possessis et arrepticijs, per euangelicas etiam historias'.

92 Despite the preponderance of female witches elsewhere, in France, at least in the early period, the ratio seems to be less skewed. Alfred Soman 1992, p. x, also found this to be the case in the *écrous* of the Conciergerie du Palais, the prison of the Parlement of Paris. He also found that very few accused sorcerers were killed.

93 The sorcerers' social position appears in some ways similar to that of the Jews studied by David Nirenberg 1996. He argues that outbreaks of violence against Jews were deeply embedded in specific social, political, and ideological conflicts that were locally based. In fact, Nirenberg suggests that coexistence was predicated on just such occasional outbreaks of violence, which could dissolve the tensions of everyday life. This argument casts new light onto considerations of 'othering', violence, and community, suggesting that persecution did not intend to purify, but to enable cohabitation. It is also worth noting, as Miri Rubin 1999 points out, that violent episodes against the Jews were not only localized and particular, but also manipulated and comprehended through narrative constructions.

94 AN JJ 199 fo 276 no 441: 'fut fort trouble de son sens et entendement criant a haulte voix comme incensee soy voulant gecter par les fenestres en la rue'.

help her. Upset about his wife's continued frenzy, Jehan Sommet began asking his 'neighbors and other people'[95] where this illness could come from, and if they knew of any possible remedy. The response, which was presented as universal, rather than attributed to one particular source, was that his wife had been poisoned by an old, 90-year-old woman in the town, named either Guillaume or Guillemete de Pigeules called Turlateuse, 'held and reputed to be a great sorcerer and a bad woman'.[96] The helpful, but anonymous, voices of Jehan Sommet's 'neighbors and other people' further informed him that only Turlateuse could provide a remedy for her poisons, and that he would have to ask the sorcerer 'nicely' (*doulcement*) to heal his wife. If Turlateuse refused, Jehan's advisors continued, he should 'warm the soles of her feet', because on other occasions, she had healed people of similar poisons and illnesses because of threats and beatings.[97]

Armed with this helpful advice, Jehan Sommet and two of his wife's brothers, Hugues Vachon and Jehan Cavart, went to the home of Turlateuse on the ninth of August, two months after his wife had first begun to exhibit these symptoms. The three men asked Turlateuse to help Jehan Sommet's wife by healing her or providing an antidote to the poisons, but, according to the letter, she refused to do so. Naturally, they proceeded to apply a hot iron to her feet in an effort to force her to help them, adding in a few beatings around her neck with a stick. When Turlateuse remained obstinate in her refusal to help them, they departed, each one back to his own home. However, two days later, Jehan Sommet's wife worsened, becoming more frenzied than before. In his anger, Jehan Sommet called together his four closest friends, the same two brothers of his wife and two other men, Jehan Grasser and Pierre Jobert, and informed them that, to heal his wife, they were going to take Turlateuse out of her home that night and burn her feet. When one of his henchmen protested that perhaps Turlateuse's neighbors would bring them to justice for breaking into her house, Jehan Sommet replied that all her neighbors knew she was a bad woman, and would not meddle with them. He returned home to his sick wife, who was being watched by several neighbors, but his friends went to Turlateuse's home, where they found her 'naked' in her bed. They took her to a nearby churchyard, where they beat her with sticks so hard that she fell on the ground, and kept beating her until she told them Jehan Sommet's wife had recovered. One of the perpetrators went to Jehan Sommet's house to verify Turlateuse's

95 AN JJ 199 fo 276 no 441: 'a ses voisins et a autres personnes'.

96 AN JJ 199 fo 276 no 441: 'tenus et repputee estre grant sorciere et mauvaise femme'.

97 AN JJ 199 fo 276 no 441: 'luy chauffast les solles des piez'.

statement, where he found the woman's health improved. Jehan went to the churchyard and found Turlateuse lying still on the ground. He claimed later he was very angry to find that his friends had beaten the sorcerer so badly, and he insisted she be carried back to her home. One of his friends did so, but, finding the door locked, left her, still naked, on the doorstep, where she was found the next morning, dead.

In some cases, mad people themselves, rather than only their relatives, were involved in gathering together a posse of like-minded individuals to 'interrogate' a renowned sorcerer. Guille Moler, in his letter of remission from 1452, claimed he was pulled out of bed one Saturday evening at eight o'clock by Jaures Menefevre, who asked Guille to join him and Thogny de la Villate, who was waiting for them with Beguite Clote. There is no indication in the letter of any kin relationship between these three men. Beguite 'as it is said, had ensorcelled the said Thogny and made him languish in a certain illness by virtue of certain evil arts such that he had lost his good, natural senses and that he was out of good memory'.[98] Interestingly, Thogny, despite believing Beguite was the cause of his illness, had asked her to heal him, which she promised to do but never managed. When the three men confronted her with rigorous words, she refused to help Thogny, so they beat her with 'little' sticks until she finally agreed to heal him. According to Guille's letter, the three men then left her alone, and she decided to sleep under a tree, where she may have taken cold, or possibly been more severely injured than they had thought, because she died the same night and her body was found under the tree the next morning.

Guitiere des Ganes' letter of remission demonstrates the general fear of sorcerers. Guitiere was eighteen years old in 1469, when she became involved in what reads as a complicated and fraught household arrangement. It is unclear from the letter exactly how Guitiere was involved in the household of Remond Robin, but it seems likely she was a servant. Remond Robin was married to Michelle Peronne, and the couple lived with their daughter, Jehanne Robine, and her husband, Roger Colmet, who had come into the household originally as a servant. Remond Robin became aware that his wife did not take good care of her children, and became so angry about it that he ended up bedridden from illness. Michelle Peronne moved out of their communal home. At this point in the narrative, Guitiere was

98 AN JJ 181 fo 67v no 123: 'come len disoit avoit ensorcele ledit thogny et le fait languer en certaine maladie par vertu de certain mauvais art tellement quil en avoit perdu son bon sens naturel et quil en estoit hors de bonne memoire'.

reintroduced, arguing that she did not dare to do anything to anger Michelle Peronne because she believed Michelle had caused her brother to become mad by making him eat the brains of a cat. The narrative suggests some intervention by a notary questioning this statement, because the letter's flow was interrupted to explain that 'the said supplicant presumed this because this Michelle had, around the feast of Easter last, treated the brain of a cat and given it to her daughter to give to the said Roger to bring him so that he would become mad'.[99] The madness of her brother worked as an insurance of her cooperation, according to Guitiere, so that she had no choice but to join Michelle Peronne and Jehanne Robine when they went to Roger Colmet's house and murdered him in his bed. According to the letter, Michelle Peronne had already confessed to all of her own crimes, and had exonerated Guitiere and Jehanne.

These cases involving sorcery, much like those that mention failed pilgrimages, demonstrate the desire for action on the part of the family and relatives of the mad. They were not willing to merely accept madness as a just punishment from God or as a natural illness that had to be endured. Their search for a solution to the problem that madness posed reached outwards, to things in their control. Many scholars writing about witchcraft have considered the cathartic value of the witch as a scapegoat for larger problems in the community.[100] Rather than target the mad to prevent such problematic crimes, some communities chose to protect them, reintegrating mad people and, in the process, channeling that potential towards recognized and 'renowned' outsiders.

IV. Understanding the Mad

In most cases, madness was recognized as an illness with no clear external cause. Faced with a family member whose actions were so disruptive, many narratives tried to understand what might motivate a mad person to commit a crime, focusing on the misinterpretation of circumstances that might cause them to react inappropriately. These ranged from simple or complex misunderstandings in the moment to long term refusals to accept the truth of a situation.

99 AN JJ 196 fo 72 no 127: 'ce presupposist ladite suppliant par ce que icelle michelle environ la feste de pasques dernier ladite michelle avoit trait la cervelle dun chat et baille a sa fille pour bailler donner audit roger amena affin quil devensist fol'.

100 Briggs 1989; Briggs 1996; Roper 2004; Roper 1994.

Guillaume Audoyn, whose case is briefly described in Chapter One, fell off a ladder and hit his head in 1403. Guillaume had been considered an idiot, out of his senses and memory, for two years when he killed his wife while loading manure onto a cart. Believing she was mocking him with her movements 'because he was stupid and idiotic through lack of sense, angered and incensed', he knocked her over with his pitchfork and hit her several times, then drove away with the cart.[101] When he returned and found his wife dead, he was surprised and angry, believing someone else had done it. This description of his actions after murdering his wife further indicated his disturbed mind, since he did not remember killing her and therefore did not flee the scene. The composers of Guillaume Audoyn's letter constructed a logical narrative to explain why he would murder his wife and why he did not react to her death in an expected way. His type of permanent stupidity caused by an accident was not considered particularly serious until he committed this crime, since he was still capable of working and had managed to do so for two years without any adverse effects. Nevertheless, his lack of comprehension was dangerous, because he misinterpreted his wife's actions as mocking. His general lack of sense had much more serious repercussions, due to his inability to recognize his wife's actions as those of a woman lifting manure into a cart.

While Guillaume Audoyn's misinterpretation was relatively simple, Jehan Massetirer, who suffered from melancholy in 1394, seemed to develop a complex theological misunderstanding. Having fallen ill from a 'natural sickness', Jehan had a candle placed in his hand, indicating he was on his deathbed and receiving extreme unction. It was after he had received the sacrament for the end of life that Jehan Massetirer's natural illness progressed into a state of madness. The madness acted as an extension of the illness, increasing the severity of it and causing him 'because of melancholy of the head' to get up from his sickbed and leave the house.[102] He walked down to the river, planning to drown himself. However, his wife, who was instrumental in seeking the letter of remission, which responded to the supplication of Jehan Massetirer's 'wife and close family',[103] followed him. With the help of two passersby,

101 AN JJ 160 fo 70v no 91, edited in Guérin 1909, vol. 7, pp. 80–82: 'pour ce qu'il estoit sourt et ydiot par non sens, yré et courroucé de ce'.

102 AN JJ 146 fo 65rv no 129: 'maladie naturele'; 'cathandelle en la main cuidant que il deust trespassee vi depuis le lendemain'; 'par merancolie de teste'.

103 AN JJ 146 fo 65rv no 129: 'humble supplicacion de la femme et amis charnelz de feu Jehan Massetirer'.

she pulled him out of the water and asked why he had allowed himself to fall into the river. Jehan Massetirer, 'full of fatuity or of sickness', responded 'that they had sinned greatly in taking him out and that he needed to die'.[104] Although they were able to get Jehan Massetirer back to his house and into his bed, he merely waited until he had been left alone with a neighbor before hitting her over the head and throwing himself into the well to drown.

Jehan Massetirer's desire for death, interpreted by his family as madness, is evocative of an extreme literalism. He 'needed to die', perhaps because he had already received extreme unction. While the assurance that a suicide had been reconciled with God before going mad and seeking death could have been intended merely as a mitigating factor in his or her favor, in this letter it is given an unexpected weight through Jehan Massetirer's speech. The composers of his remission letter opened the possibility that it was the sacrament itself that ultimately led to his death. Interestingly, a similar letter from 1420 did not include madness as a possible reason for someone to commit suicide after receiving extreme unction. Jehan du Puy was so ill that he had made his will, confessed, and received extreme unction before cutting his own throat. The composers of his letter explained his actions by suggesting he committed suicide because of 'temptation of the enemy, because of the oppression of his illness, or from some other cause',[105] but they did not suggest madness or a literal interpretation of the sacrament as an excuse.

In complicated ways, madness was seen as potentially caused by powerful emotions. As the letters about loss of property during the war indicate, grief about loss was a powerful emotion that could cause people to act in unexpected ways. Some remission letter composers went even further, providing explanations that explored the inner workings of a person's mind, focusing on a perceived inability to fulfill familial and household roles, guilt, or familial conflicts as catalysts for madness. While some of these emotions, such as jealousy, anger, and despair, are actually named (*jalousie*, *courroucie*, and *desespere*), others are described in great detail, without being given a specific term to define them. Extremes of emotion were described as moments of inner conflict that could lead to madness.[106]

104 AN JJ 146 fo 65rv no 129: 'le qel plain de fatuite ou de maladie quel avion respondi quils avoient fait grant pechie de lentue hors et que il ydeuoit mourir'.

105 AN JJ 171 fo 94v no 156: 'pour ce que par temptacion de lennemj pour cause de loppression de maladie ou autrement il sest coppes la gorge en commectant homicide de lui mesme'.

106 For more on this topic, see my essay, Pfau 2010a.

Barbara Rosenwein contends that historians should 'worry' about emotions in history, particularly in the Middle Ages, and offers the term 'emotional communities' to help

> uncover systems of feeling: what these communities (and the individuals within them) define and assess as valuable or harmful to them; the evaluations that they make about others' emotions; the nature of the affective bonds between people that they recognize; and the modes of emotional expression that they expect, encourage, tolerate, and deplore.[107]

The question of emotions and of enacting emotional responses has been 'worrying' medievalists partly in response to Johan Huizinga's image of a Middle Ages filled with 'childish emotions' and Norbert Elias's suggestion that the sixteenth century saw the development of the 'civilizing process' that caused people to repress and restrain their emotions.[108] Stephen Jaeger's response to Elias moved the civilizing moment back to the tenth century,[109] but more recent work on emotions in the Middle Ages has shifted focus from the 'civilizing process' to the ways medieval people used emotional displays for particular goals. Stephen White claims that eleventh-, twelfth-, and thirteenth-century emotions, particularly of anger, were 'highly conventionalized and socially generated', and were enacted for specific political strategies.[110] Daniel Smail similarly notes that 'men and women in Marseille and elsewhere in medieval Europe found it useful to have or autosuggest states of anger and hatred and, perhaps, learned how to perform fictive emotional states if the subcortex refused to cooperate'.[111] Remission letters suggest, however, that while certain emotional displays were considered appropriate and even politically expedient, an excessive display of emotion could be perceived as irrational madness.[112]

107 Rosenwein 2002, p. 842.
108 Elias 1978; Huizinga 1954.
109 Jaeger 1985.
110 Stephen D. White 1998, p. 150.
111 Smail 2003, p. 244.
112 It is, of course, necessary to be cautious when discussing the connections between emotions and rationality in the Middle Ages. After all, the Cartesian separation between the emotional and the rational, and thus the body and the mind, had not yet been formulated. However, perturbation of the 'passions' was one of Galen's six non-naturals, which he understood as causing disruptions in the ideal humoral balance of the individual, and thus as potentially damaging to the senses. See Siraisi 1990, p. 101. In addition, medieval legal treatises, such as Albertanus of Brescia's *Liber consolationis et consilii*, composed in 1246, believed that extreme emotion could lead to madness (here called *furiosus*), and sought to temper such emotional excess in the quest

In 1460, Guillaume Sunoneau, at the age of thirty-five, composed a letter to the king asking for remission for a crime committed in his youth, some seventeen or eighteen years before. Guillaume explained that at that time 'from temptation of the enemy or otherwise' he had had carnal relations, 'once with a mare and five or six times with a cow'.[113] It is worth pointing out that, if Guillaume was correct about his chronology, he would have been twelve or thirteen when he committed this crime, and thus not of an age where he could have been held legally responsible for his actions.[114] Guillaume gives no excuse for his actions other than the temptation of the devil, and madness does not appear in his life until long afterwards, when he finds himself unable to forget his 'sin'.[115] His feelings of displeasure and anger towards himself for having committed crimes, 'knowing that these were enormous and detestable',[116] served as a catalyst for madness. While these particular sentiments only appear in this letter, they are worth analyzing because this is also the only letter that deals with the connection between sin and madness. None of the letters of remission suggest that sin was a direct cause of madness. Although religious ideas are present in these letters, it is clear that the concept that madness only happened to the sinful did not loom large in the minds of the composers of remission letters.[117] The linkage of sin and madness would have been familiar to a medieval audience from the Biblical story of Nebuchadnezzar, whose hubris led God to punish him with madness. However, in Guillaume's letter he explained that his sin caused guilt which led to madness. He did not perceive his madness as a direct punishment from God for his sinful behavior.

Although Guillaume confessed and received absolution from the church, he was never pursued by the king's justice, and therefore he believed he had

to prevent impulsive vengeance. Jacqueline Van Leeuwen 2005 discusses the translation of Albertanus' treatise into Dutch. For an interesting exploration of the development of the study of emotions, see Deploige 2005.

113 AN JJ 190 fo 33 no 64: 'par temptacion de lennemy ou autrement habita par une foiz avec une jument et par cinq ou six foiz avec une vache'.

114 The age of responsibility, and of consent (which is clearly relevant here), was twelve for girls and fourteen for boys.

115 AN JJ 190 fo 33 no 64: 'pechir'.

116 AN JJ 190 fo 33 no 64: 'sachant iceulx estre enormes et detestables'.

117 See Doob 1974. See also Fritz 1992, pp. 165–191, for a discussion of the sermon literature and theoretical literature that presents this argument. It is interesting that sermons did not make much of an impact in this case.

not sufficiently paid for his crime.[118] In his remission letter, he explained that

> for the grand displeasure and anger that he had towards himself for the horror and infamy of this and also for the great sin that he felt he had committed in this case towards God our creator, [he] entered into such a melancholy and displeasure that he was alienated and troubled in his good sense and understanding such that he had two or three times despaired and wanted to kill and drown himself, and afterwards he, thus troubled and altered, went before the eyes of the justice of Osain and of his own movement, without being constrained nor accused but liberally and of his frank will told and confessed having committed the said acts in the manner in which it is here above declared and for this cause was taken and constituted prisoner.[119]

Guillaume was driven into a melancholy madness because of his feelings of horror and anger against himself about the sin he had committed in his youth. He was unable to assuage his self-directed anger through the mechanisms offered by the church, and so he turned himself in to the secular law, taking himself 'before the eyes of the justice of Osain' to confess publicly to the government's representatives. His decision to turn himself in to the officers of the law was described in the letter as part of his madness. The idea that a desire to be punished for committing a crime was evidence of a lack of reason appeared in at least two other letters,[120] suggesting that it was considered rational to try to avoid punishment. Guillaume's troubling and suicidal desire to 'kill and drown himself' was transferred into a desire for

118 See Mansfield 1995 for a discussion of guilt and confession, particularly pages 35–36, where she talks about cases where guilt prompted confession, and page 81 where she notes a sermon exemplum in which a woman commits suicide because of her inability to confess to having consented to her mother's murder. Note also Texier 2001, p. 490, where he links the narrative frame of remission letters to the system of religious confession in terms of temptation and repentance.

119 AN JJ 190 fo 33 no 64: 'pour le grant desplaisir et courroux quil en avoit en soy mesmes pour horreur et infame diceulx et aussi pour le grant pechir quil sentoit a ceste cause avoir commis envers dieu notre createur est entre en une telle merancolie et desplaisance quil sen est aliene et trouble en son bon sens et entendement et tellement quil a este par deux ou trois foiz en voye de desespoir et de fait sest voulu occire et noyer et apres lui estant ainsi trouble et altere sen est ale devant les yeus de la justice du lieu de osain et de son propre mouvement sans contraincte ne accusacion leut a liberalment et de sa franche voulente dit et confesse avoir commis lesdis cas en la maniere quil est cy dessus declare et a ceste cause fut mis et constitue prisonnier'.

120 AN JJ 188 fo 10 no 15 (in 1458) and AN JJ 188 fo 81 no 160 (in 1459). The former is edited in Guérin 1909, vol. 10, pp. 92–94.

an equally suicidal but more public expurgation of his crime through the mechanisms of secular law. Indeed, it seems that Guillaume, or the notary who helped him compose his letter, had internalized the discourse of the execution of convicted criminals as public spectacle. Ultimately, however, since Guillaume himself sought this remission, he must have changed his mind about his desire for full punishment under the law.[121] Perhaps the reading of his confessional letter of remission by the local justice was a sufficiently public ritual to expiate his guilt, or perhaps Guillaume had recovered his 'sanity' while in prison.

Unfounded jealousy of spouses suspected of infidelity appeared quite often in the remission letters, as a catalyst for despair and suicide and sometimes as a cause for murder. Even when there were grounds for jealousy, these people acted on their emotions in ways that were considered excessive and unacceptable. By attempting to comprehend these cases in terms of madness, the family and relatives could reconcile these actions and reintegrate into the community those who survived these moments of rupture. Symonnet de la Dert, called Bridalet, fell into jealousy in 1394 because of 'false reports of women or other people' which had accused his wife of infidelity and his daughter (of marriageable age) of fornication.[122] As a result of his great jealousy he 'became thus as if completely furious and insensible and stopped doing his work and became idle and for hours was in such a state that he did not know what he said nor what he did'.[123] Symonnet de la Dert's entire household and community suffered, since he was incapable of working as a result of his jealousy, which (according to the letter composed on behalf of the wife and daughter) was entirely unfounded. He beat his wife and daughter, and then ran away to the woods for two days. After returning to his home, he still refused to work, forcing his wife and daughter to seek employment outside the house and leave him alone, when 'being in his said fury, by temptation of the enemy, he hanged himself'.[124]

In a similar case from 1426, Jehannette Maillart committed suicide because she was 'often weakened in her understanding, and as if furious, as much from drinking too much, in which she felt herself drowning, as

121 Since all remission letters are for crimes punishable by death, a desire to receive remission indicates that Guillaume Sunoneau was no longer feeling suicidal.

122 AN JJ 146 fo 83v no 162: 'faulx rappors de femmes ou autres personnes'. It is not entirely clear who the 'other people' described might be – men, one hazards.

123 AN JJ 146 fo 83v no 162: 'devint ainsi comme tout furieux et insensible et delaissoit afaire son labour et estoit oiseux et par heures estoit en cel estoit que il ne savoit quil disoit ne quil faisoit'.

124 AN JJ 146 fo 83v no 162: 'estant en sa dicte fuerosite par temptacion de lannemj se pendi'.

from suspicion of jealousy that she had against her said husband without cause'.[125] In this case, Jehannette Maillart's madness was attributable either to her drinking[126] or to her jealousy of her husband. Neither her husband, who was seeking a letter of remission for her, nor the royal notary, who helped compose the letter, considered it necessary to determine which was the ultimate source. The important point from the perspective of the letter composers was her lack of understanding, either due to her illness or to her jealousy, which made her lack culpability for any action she might take. In both these cases, the surviving family members insisted the jealousy was unwarranted, establishing their own innocence in the sordid suicides. Rather, the suicide victims became the active parties, causing their own deaths, both through their incapacity to understand the truth (that their spouses were faithful) and through the crimes that their jealousy and madness drove them to commit. In Symonnett's case, he would not have been given the opportunity to kill himself if his madness had not caused him to become idle and forced his wife and daughter to leave him alone in the house. Similarly, Jehannette's illness might have had as large a role in her ultimate death as her suspicion of her husband.

A third narrative of jealousy played out to a very different ending. It began with the same basic storyline. In 1425, Simon Rogate became jealous of his wife, who, he believed, was having an affair with Huguenin Baulion, the son of their neighbor, whom it had been rumored she might marry before her marriage to Simon. However, from that point the narrative departed from the familiar tale of mistaken jealousy. Rather, Simon Rogate actually caught his wife and Huguenin together in suspicious circumstances and confronted her. According to the letter, their confrontation turned into an argument, during which Simon's wife informed him that she 'would have preferred to marry [Huguenin] than [Simon]' and admitted she had had carnal relations with Huguenin.[127] This news 'placed [Simon] in even greater suspicion, anger and melancholy', emotions that ultimately led him, several days later, to beat his wife.[128] Though he explained in the

125 AN JJ 173 fo 188v no 392, edited mistakenly as JJ 175 no 392 in Longnon 1878, p. 208: 'souvent ebetée de son entendement, et comme furieuse, tant par trop boire dont elle se sentoit delegier, et par souspeçon de jalousie qu'elle avoit sans cause contre son dit mary'.
126 Karla Taylor, in a personal communication in February 2006, pointed out that this description seems to fit the illness of hydromania, an excessive need for water. The text is ambiguous, and may refer to drinking too much water or to becoming drunk, but either way her madness appeared connected to her drinking according to the composers of the letter.
127 AN JJ 173 fo 168 no 349: 'lamast mieulx avoir espouse que icellui suppliant'.
128 AN JJ 173 fo 168 no 349: 'mis en plusgrant souspecon courrouz et melancolie'.

letter he had intended the beating merely as a corrective, his wife died from it, and he was forced to seek remission for murder. Jealousy could drive people to a violent madness that was directed outwards, as well as towards themselves.

Marguerite Bouchart was around forty years old in 1489 when her husband decided (against Marguerite's will) that they would move away from the village they had lived in for most of their married life. Marguerite explained that because 'it was such a strange thing for her to make a new household, she became as if completely out of her good sense and understanding, and being in this grief and displeasure', she tried to prevent people from moving her things out of her house.[129] In what at first seems to be a rather petty act of defiance, Marguerite took a container of onions from the cart of moveable goods, threw most of them in the water, and cut up some others to eat right away. Marguerite's husband responded by yelling at her, and then began to beat her. She, 'not knowing what she was doing', stabbed him with the knife she had been using to cut the onions, giving him a wound that proved fatal.[130]

In many respects, Marguerite's remission letter reads like those of other domestic disputes that do not mention madness as a possible reason for a wife to kill her husband. Her husband was beating her while she was holding a knife in her hand for legitimate purposes, and before her husband died, he had forgiven her for the act.[131] Nevertheless, the decision to explain her actions as rooted in a temporary lack of sense and understanding, such that she 'did not know what she was doing',[132] granted a particularity to her crime. Marguerite's actions were not merely those of a woman upset at leaving her home, but the actions of a woman whose distress at a situation she could not control had driven her out of her mind. The discourse of madness in this remission letter, in a sense, provided a space within which Marguerite could act upon her emotions, of sorrow and frustration, in a violent way. Her momentary experience of being 'out of her senses' was considerably more transitory than the madness of other people who appear in remission letters. However, the way the discourse of madness could be deployed even in such

129 AN JJ 220 fo 52v no 90: 'quil lui estoit chose fort estrange faire nouveau mesnage quelle en fut comme tout hors debon sens et entendement et elle estant en ceste douleur et desplaisir'.

130 AN JJ 220 fo 52v no 90: 'ne savoit quelle faisoit'.

131 See Davis 1987, pp. 77–110, where she discusses the themes of accidental violence provoked by a beating in stories of women killing their husbands. Although she is addressing a later period, the themes are already present in these letters. See also Gauvard 1991, vol. 2, p. 573. Gauvard argues that domestic violence accounts for only two percent of the letters of remission. Interestingly, the percentage is much higher within cases citing madness as a reason for the crime.

132 AN JJ 220 fo 52v no 90: 'quelle ne savoit quelle faisoit'.

a weak case suggests the strength of the conceptual connection between family strife, emotion, and madness.

Madness was often seen as caused by family situations that could not be controlled. Phote, probably short for Philippote, Brumel, the widow of a knight, had a young daughter named Marguerite for whom she had arranged an advantageous marriage in 1379. Unfortunately, Marguerite had been impregnated by Phot, most likely a diminutive of Philippot, le Roy, their carter. When Phote discovered that her daughter was pregnant, and by an employee, she 'was much marvelously grieved and astonished because she had believed that her said daughter was a good girl'.[133] According to the letter, the birth of the baby caused Phote to lose her reason, and

> then the said Phote as if entirely despairing and angered by this event, still remembering how her said daughter was promised by marriage to a knight of the country, said to the said Phot, tempted by the enemy and as if out of her senses, that he should take the said infant and that he should carry it with her and that he should never talk about it. So the said Phot took the infant and carried it with the said Phote up to the place called the Lodges near the said town of Mareygny and they found a well nearby into the which well the said Phote, thus angered and insane [*forsenée*] as has been said, said to the said Phot that he should throw the said infant and forthwith the said Phot threw this infant into the said well.[134]

The narrative presented a mother who was thwarted in her plans to support her daughter through an advantageous marriage, and who was driven mad by despair and anger. Her accomplice, Phot, moved to another town, where he was found and brought to justice, at which point Phote feared she had been implicated in the crime. Indeed, Phote herself seemed to believe that her decision to kill the baby was wrong, since she and her daughter immediately went into self-imposed exile before seeking a letter of remission to exonerate

133 AN JJ 114 fo 116v no 236: 'fu moult merveilliee dolente et esbahie car elle cuidoit sa dite fille estre bonne pucelle'.

134 AN JJ 114 fo 116v no 236: 'lors la dite phote comme toute desesperee et courrociee dudit cas encore soy remembrant comme sa dite fille estoit promise par mariage a un escuier du pais dist audit phot temptee de lennemj et comme hors de son sens quil preist le dit enfant et quil le portast avec elle et que jamais il ne le rapporteroient adont le dit phot print le dit enfant et le porta avec la dite phote jusques au lieu dit les loges pres de la dite ville de mareygny et trouverent un puis pres dillec dedans le quel puis la dite phote ainsi corrociee et forsenee comme dit est dist au dit phot que il y gectast le dit enfant et incontinent gecta le dit phot ycellui enfant dedans le dit puis'.

her. She explained that the decision to commit infanticide arose from her despair, causing her to become mad and take actions that, in a less stressful situation, she would never have considered.

Domestic problems had to be relatively excessive to believably provoke madness in response. For example, in a letter from 1490, Laurens de Pre explained that he had lived in a household with his wife's parents, which made for an uncomfortable domestic situation. After Laurens's wife gave birth to their first child, his mother-in-law, Marguerite Collard, conceived 'such a great hatred' for him that she decided to keep her daughter away from him, and would not allow them to sleep together.[135] This caused 'great sorrow' for Laurens.[136] When Laurens tried one night to sneak into the bed his wife was sharing with her mother, Marguerite Collard woke up and hit him on the head with a big stick. Temporarily out of his senses, he took out the knife he used to cut bread, and killed her. In this case, both an untenable situation that continued over time and a blow to the head at the moment of the crime were required to make Laurens de Pre so stunned 'that he did not know what he was doing or where he was'.[137]

Family conflicts could also become the source of a form of temporary insanity with much milder results. For example, Gernaye Pillot moved to a new town, where in 1459 he became engaged without the counsel of his father or any of his family. When he came to ask his father to help him pay for his wedding, his father refused. 'Troubled in his understanding' because of his father's refusal, Gernaye stole some cows to use to pay for his wedding.[138] Because Gernaye was not the head of a household, he was subject to his father's will. Having broken that will by becoming engaged without seeking advice, Gernaye was punished, which caused him to resort to theft, further alienating himself from his family. The letter of remission, which he sought for himself, developed the theme of a prodigal son who was spurned, rather than fêted, on his return.

Conflicts were often instigated when the mad person, like Symonnett de la Dert described above, could no longer fulfill expected household roles. For example, during her pregnancy in 1423, Jehannette Voidié believed that her husband's income would not allow them to support a third child, despite his reassurance.[139] Her family later interpreted Jehannette's feelings

135 AN JJ 221 fo 124v no 215: 'si grant hayne'.

136 AN JJ 221 fo 124v no 215: 'grant dueil'.

137 AN JJ 221 fo 124v no 215: 'quil ne savoit quil faisoit ne ou il estoit'.

138 AN JJ 188 fo 82v no 163.

139 AN JJ 172 fo 239 no 430, edited in Longnon 1878, pp. 130–133.

of insecurity as a direct cause of her madness. When she gave birth to a son, she lost her milk because of an argument she had with the lying-in maid over some linens,[140] and the baby had to be sent to a wet-nurse.[141] This sent Jehannette even further into a melancholy, during which she did not interact with her husband or her other children, telling them 'they had in her a bad mother'.[142] Jehan Lambert, her husband, repeatedly assured her that he made enough money to support their family, and then threatened to beat her if she continued to repine. She responded that she wished he would beat her to death, and proceeded to attempt to commit suicide. When her child returned from the wet-nurse, he was very sickly, and Jehannette Voidié decided to take him on a pilgrimage. On the way, she stopped for her sister, and while she was waiting, Jehannette, upset about her child's weakness, 'entered into her said melancholies and furor or lack of sense, as it is to be believed and presumed, and by temptation of the enemy threw this her infant into the well'.[143] Her sister, hearing the splash, ran back. When she told Jehannette Voidié that she was a bad mother and had drowned her baby, Jehannette denied it, insisting the baby was fine, and joining enthusiastically in the attempts to fish him out. Eventually, however, she left the scene and ran away. The letter thus describes a drastic change in behavior during this recent pregnancy that made Jehannette unrecognizable. Although the letter does not give much detail about her life before, it is clear that Jehannette's husband found her behavior baffling.

Unlike Jehannette, who was portrayed as mistaken about her husband's income, Gouyn Cluchat faced a real family crisis in 1459.[144] As noted above, his failure to protect his family was the source of his despair. When the plague arrived in their village, he moved himself, his wife, and their four

140 The period immediately following childbirth was a dangerous time, and conflicts between lying-in maids and mothers, resulting in a loss of milk or other problems with the baby, were not unusual. Indeed, a century later such conflicts were likely to result in witchcraft accusations against the lying-in maid. For more on these relationships, see Roper 1994.

141 It is clear from the text that Jehannette Voidié was expected to nurse her own child, but that the family had the resources to hire a wetnurse if necessary. Wetnursing was a relatively common practice at this time, despite a growing literature encouraging women to nurse their own babies for fear the wetnurse's milk would adversely affect the child. For an exploration of these themes as they relate to Italy, see Klapisch-Zuber 1985.

142 AN JJ 172 fo 239 no 430, edited in Longnon 1878, pp. 130-133: 'qu'ilz avoient en elle une mauvaise mere'.

143 AN JJ 172 fo 239 no 430, edited in Longnon 1878, pp. 130-133: 'entra en sesdictes melancolies et fureur ou non sens, comme il est à croire et presumer, et par temptacion de l'ennemi gecta icellui son enfant ou puys'.

144 AN JJ 188 fo 81 no 160.

young children to a neighboring town to escape from the danger. A few months later, Cluchat's wife fell ill with a fever, and he realized they were running out of provisions. Although they had left behind some flour and some wine in their village, he did not dare to return for them because of the plague. Instead, he went into a nearby city to borrow some flour or some money to support his sick wife and his children, but no one was willing to help him. After escaping from the plague, he and his family seemed likely to starve instead. This crisis made Cluchat so upset that he went to a fountain in the town, thinking in his despair to drown himself, but a woman who happened to be passing stopped to ask him what he was doing, and he was so embarrassed he left. Arriving at his house, 'as if he was out of his senses', Cluchat took an axe used for chopping wood, and hit his wife on the head with it and killed her.[145] Here the composers of the remission letter described a more evident rupture of selfhood. Gouyn Cluchat was described through most of the letter as a man who cared for his family's safety and wellbeing. He took them to a new town to escape from the plague, and went out to beg to prevent them from starving. It was only after his failure to provide for them that his identity cracked. Had his suicide attempt succeeded, he would have left his children and his sick wife to fend for themselves, which clearly does not fit his behavior pattern up to this point. His ultimate crime of killing his wife with an axe, therefore, was connected to this pattern of unacceptable behavior in the narrative.

In these cases, feelings of insecurity and a perceived inability (on the part of themselves or others) to care for their families led these people to madness and sometimes suicide attempts. Although neither Jehannette's nor Gouyn's story ended with self-murder, it is clear that their families saw a connection between their ultimate crime and their previous desire to turn their anger and fears against themselves. Family conflicts often arose due to the mad person's inability to fulfill certain expected roles. Not all the remission letters about madness set up such clear patterns of usual and unusual behaviors in the lives of the individuals they described, but the letters that did actually attempted to enter into the mad person's perception of reality to understand how the particular mad person understood the world and why he or she might therefore have committed a criminal act. Even in cases where the fears of the mad are unfounded, they are based on recognizable problems.

Remission letters give us a window into some of the methods the letter composers used to understand the crimes committed by the mad. One of the

145 AN JJ 188 fo 81 no 160: 'come hors du sens et debilite de son entendement'.

ways in which medieval families coped with these crimes was by seeking to explain them. While the actions of the mad could appear inappropriate and inexplicable to an external observer, within the context of the remission letter the composers sometimes tried to justify the crime based on the mad person's flawed perception of reality. In contrast to the philosophy of the first-century Greek physician Aretaeus, who believed that mad people saw as other people did but interpreted what they saw incorrectly,[146] remission letters seem to suggest that mad people actually experienced a different reality. From the rhetorical frame of the relatives and immediate family, the composers of these letters ultimately discussed the event from the perspective of the primary actor involved, resulting in complicated attempts to comprehend the motivations of a person perceived as mad. Thus, some letters superimposed explicable motives onto the narrative of a mad crime in an effort to force the crime to be comprehensible. Through these attempts an image of the internal viewpoint of a mad mind emerged.

Unlike the more common murders in remission letters, which took place in taverns or on the street, generally after drinking and various forms of gambling, the crimes of the mad were much more likely to take place inside the home, and often the victim was a family member. Therefore, the violence of the mad was disquieting and difficult to explain. While some letters chose to describe this violence as motiveless and unexpected, many remission letters cited common troubles, such as poverty, jealousy, and guilt, either as direct causes of madness or as the results of a mad person's flawed perception of reality. For example, in the case of Jehannette Voidié, who dropped her legitimate baby son in a well in 1423, the composers of her letter explained that during her pregnancy she had been concerned about whether the family could support another child, and that she had often spoken of herself as a bad mother.[147] These concerns, according to the composers of the letter, were completely groundless, since her husband could support another child, but Jehannette's understanding of reality was skewed.[148] Instead of suggesting that she threw her child in the well for no discernable reason, the composers of the letter tried to understand the crime. The problem was in Jehannette's flawed perception of reality, not only in terms of her inability to recognize that her family could support another child, but

146 Rosen 1968, p. 97.

147 Madness was often linked to infanticide cases where the child was legitimate, since there was no culturally recognized reason to get rid of or hide a legitimate birth.

148 AN JJ 172 fo 239 no 430, edited in Longnon 1878, pp. 130–133.

also in her belief that killing the child was a reasonable response to the crisis she supposedly perceived.

There was no single way to reconstruct the past in remission letters, and no particular narrative that acted as proof of a history of madness. Each story reconstructed the past of the individual in a way that highlighted those moments that seemed mad to the composers. In the case of Jehan de Moustier discussed in Chapter Two, his mad behavior was centered on food. The narrative of his letter confirmed his madness, arguing that it was clear from his actions and also providing a clear history of behavior that led up to the murder of his father.[149] While on the one hand this exculpated Jehan de Moustier completely, on the other it confirmed his madness to such an extent that he was only released into the care of his family on condition that he be kept chained. Jehannette Voidié's actions were described much more cautiously, whether by the choice of her relatives and close family or because of the recommendation of the royal notary. While her suicide attempts were certainly attributed to her melancholy, the language used in the remission letter suggests some doubt about what caused her to throw her child into the well. It was 'presumed' that she entered into her melancholy and frenzy, but it was not certain.[150] In the end, Jehannette Voidié was given remission on condition that she be kept in prison for fifteen days on bread and water, and that she pay for fifty masses to be sung for her dead child, a punishment that seems more appropriate for someone who was in fact guilty of committing a crime, rather than someone who was not considered responsible for her own actions.

Jehan Lambert could support another child, but there were people whose fears were not so imaginary. Gouyn Cluchat, stuck between plague and starvation, was unable to support his family.[151] The composers of his remission letter emphasized the fact that Gouyn Cluchat was unable to find help in the region, and that the murder of his wife was caused by extreme provocation. Unlike Jehannette, Cluchat was fully aware of what he had done, and went out of the house to find some neighbors so he could tell them he had just killed his wife. Indeed, he went even further, traveling to the nearby city of Combronde and demanding they put him to death for his crime. To the family members composing his letter of remission and even to the officers in Combronde, his desire to be hanged was further proof of his madness. However, the composers of his letter explained, since

149 AN JJ 118 fo 18v no 18.

150 AN JJ 172 fo 239 no 430, edited in Longnon 1878, pp. 130–133: 'comme il est à croire et presumer'.

151 AN JJ 188 fo 81 no 160.

the officers did not dare to proceed against him he was likely to remain in prison indefinitely, unless the king stepped in to pardon him. This letter, like many others, leaves us with no clear picture of the ultimate fate of the madman. He was released from prison on the authority of the king, and with no conditions such as keeping him chained up or under guard. His family seemed to believe his release would prevent his children from becoming beggars, but they provided no hint about what would be done to cope with his extreme melancholy and his desire to be punished for his crime.

In these cases, there are distinct understandings of madness at work. With Jehannette, her lack of knowledge of having committed the crime demonstrated to her family that she was not in her right mind when she did it.[152] In this case, her inability to recognize the results of her actions while mad meant she did not act with intent, although the fact that she was required to pay for masses for her baby's soul suggests there was some question about whether she nevertheless deserved to be punished. Jehan de Moustier was also unable to recognize his crime. When he was told he had killed his father, he responded that 'he was only my father according to whispers', which suggests he was denying his own identity.[153] In contrast, Gouyn Cluchat's admission of guilt and, further, his active desire to be punished for his crime, was cited by his family and by the officers at Combronde as a clear indication of his insanity.[154] In his insistence on guilt and punishment, the composers of his remission letter dealt with the concept of irrational behavior. Unlike the crime itself, which could be comprehended due to his flawed perception of reality, the decision to seek punishment for that crime was seen as irrational.

Moments of emotional upheaval in these letters often centered on conflicts between family members that caused one of them to become mad. Discord generally arose around questions of power dynamics within the family. The narratives built on points of tension between the familial hierarchy on the one hand and the desires of the family members to create space for their own autonomy on the other. While the disruptive response of the family member who struck out against the hierarchy was clearly considered unacceptable by the rest of the family, the label of madness opened up the possibility

152 Guillaume Audoyn was also unable to remember that he had beaten his wife in AN JJ 160 fo 70v no 91, edited in Guérin 1909, pp. 80–82.

153 AN JJ 118 fo 18v no 18: 'il dist que il nestoit son pere que dans oreille'.

154 This is also the case for Guillaume Sunoneau, who committed bestiality and chose to turn himself in to the local officials because of his guilt. See AN JJ 190 fo 33 no 64 (in 1460).

of resistance to the hierarchy while nevertheless forcing that resistance, ultimately, to be controlled and defused. These narratives described moments of rupture, where the accepted familial hierarchy was overturned, but only momentarily. By understanding these ruptures as moments of madness, the texts allowed for reconciliation and the reintegration of the recovered mad person into his or her expected position.

The brief life narratives encapsulated within remission letters conceal much about their protagonists. These crimes are told from only one perspective, that of the criminal, or in some cases of those taking the criminal's part. It is not possible to trace these crimes to their source and discover more about the community where they were committed, or find dissenting voices that could clarify the details of the case or shed light on alternative narratives about the crimes or about those who committed them. The mad people described in these letters disappeared from the public record after remission was granted. What did the family and community actually do once the mad person was released from prison? What was the long-term effect of the admission of guilt and madness on the individuals and on their communities? Answers to these questions, and many others, remain tantalizingly out of reach.

Nevertheless, these letters reveal important details about how madness was understood and what kinds of actions were taken on behalf of those considered mad. Madness, conceived as an inability to understand the world and particularly the rules, explicit and implicit, that governed human interactions, revealed the instability of communities on all levels. However, despite the medieval 'persecuting society',[155] mad people were not exiled from their communities as a result of the threat they posed. Rather, even after committing crimes, they could be reintegrated into their families and communities. The very ties they had ruptured were reconstructed through the narratives of these remission letters, as the letter composers sought to place mad people at the center of communal responsibility and concern.

The crimes of the mad, as narrated in remission letters, departed so radically from accepted norms of behavior that they made the reintegration of the guilty especially difficult. Nevertheless, remission letters sought in their narratives to reconstruct the very bonds ruptured through these crimes, not only in their hopes for the future, but also in their depictions of the past. In this way they constructed an 'imagined community' that was significantly more positive than the community in which they actually lived.

155 Moore 1987.

Conclusions

A set of four remission letters all dealing with the same crime appear in the chancery records for 1424 and 1425.[1] It is not a story about madness itself, but one that offers insight into how the discourse of madness was deployed and how multiple levels of community were constructed. In these four letters sent to the king, a number of residents of a town in the diocese of Bayeux explained to the English government of France how it came to pass that they had banded together to attack two English men in November of 1417, shortly after Henry V's army had overtaken Caen. No one could understand these strangers, who had decided to lodge at Guillaume le Paumier's *hôtel*. When the two men started to gather together the Paumiers's goods, Alips, Guillaume le Paumier's wife, left the *hôtel* seeking help, and a group of townspeople returned with her and killed the two men.

Their requests for remission were written against the background of national events. In the seven years between 1417, when the act was committed, and 1424, when remission was sought, the political landscape in France had shifted, in part due to repercussions from the king's madness. Charles VI had died in 1422, leaving political confusion and civil war dividing the realm. The dead king's son, Charles, had been officially disinherited, and controlled only southern France. His grandson, Henry, the heir according to the Treaty of Troyes, was just a baby, and with the aid of an English regent and the duke of Burgundy, held Paris and northern France. In such a divisive moment, fundamental questions about the very constitution of the French realm, French identity, and the relationship between the French and the English were at stake. The political situation was so complex in part because of the king's madness, which had left his legacy, shaped through the Treaty of Troyes, open to question.

As these four remission letters demonstrate, this confusion of loyalties on the level of the realm had repercussions in local communities. With an English king on the throne, actions that might in other contexts have appeared simply as a

1 AN JJ 173 fo 22v no 44; AN JJ 173 fo 88 no 170; AN JJ 173 fo 88v no 171; and AN JJ 173 fo 89v no 172.

Pfau, A., *Medieval Communities and the Mad: Narratives of Crime and Mental Illness in Late Medieval France.* Taylor & Francis Group, 2021
DOI: 10.5117/9789462983359_CONCL

commendable and heroic defense of the village against enemies of the realm, were suddenly construed as the murder of loyal soldiers and subjects of the king. These conflicts over changing identities and shifting boundaries between enemy and friend were relatively common in this period, and a number of remission letters reflect discomfort and uncertainty on a local level, caused by political events. This series of letters moves beyond the general acknowledgement of alternating loyalties, however, considering problems of linguistic differences, communal defense, and the long-term fears that such shifts engender.

Robert le Panomer's letter was recorded in the chancery in December of 1424, and was the first remission letter sought by members of this community in reference to the death of the two strangers.[2] The three other letters relating to this crime were all recorded consecutively in June of 1425, and appear to have been composed in consultation with each other. Indeed, these three letters are practically word for word exact replicas of each other. The first of these was composed on behalf of Guillaume and Alips le Paumier,[3] who were pardoned together as a married couple. The two others were for Robin Germain[4] and Jehan Germain,[5] perhaps brothers or a father and son, though their relationship to each other was not specified in the letters. These three identical letters with slight alterations in reference to the particular supplicant involved reveal the careful construction that went into these crime narratives. In the essentials they do not diverge significantly from Robert le Panomer's earlier version, but their narrative is more cautious and considered.

It is tempting to speculate about the exchange of information once Robert le Panomer returned to Normandy with his letter of remission. Guillaume and Alips le Paumier and Robin and Jehan Germain all claimed they had been hiding 'secretly', supported by their neighbors and relatives in the area, for the past seven years. Two possibilities can be imagined. One is that, with Robert le Panomer's letter of remission, the horizon opened for these four fugitives. Here was proof that the English occupiers would not execute them for their crime, but that Henry, like the King of France he claimed to be, would, of his grace and mercy, pardon them. Alternatively, Robert le Panomer's return with a royal pardon might have initiated a legal case against his accomplices, since remission for one participant in a crime did not guarantee remission for the others.[6] Regardless, it is likely that Robert le Panomer's remission

2 AN JJ 173 fo 22v no 44.

3 AN JJ 173 fo 88 no 170.

4 AN JJ 173 fo 88v no 171.

5 AN JJ 173 fo 89v no 172.

6 Esther Cohen notes this, although the case she discusses involves people who received remission for crimes for which their accomplices had already been executed. Cohen 1993.

letter for this case spurred the others to seek their own. The distance from Paris to the diocese of Bayeux, where their village was located, is around 260 kilometers (160 miles). There was plenty of time between Robert le Panomer's return, probably some time in late December or early January, and the trip to Paris in May or June by the other four remission seekers. They could get the story straight, ensure that the details matched and that nothing they said had the potential to backfire once they acquired remission.

The first letter, written on behalf of Robert le Panomer, claimed that two strangers arrived in town, 'speaking a strange language that they had never heard and they did not know whether they were Bretons, English, Scottish or other peoples'.[7] The letter is a narrative constructing Robert le Panomer's innocence. The men were speaking an incomprehensible language, so no one knew they were English, and, perhaps more significantly, no one knew what they were doing. They were the first aggressors. According to Robert le Panomer's letter, the strangers had threatened the Paumiers by hitting them both several times with the flat of their swords, and gathered all the Paumier's goods together, planning to steal them in the morning. As if that was not enough to exonerate him, even Alips's decision to call on her neighbors for aid was not done with the intention of attacking the two strangers, but only in a state of temporary madness brought on by fear, loss, and possibly pain, since she had already been beaten by the strangers' swords. According to Robert le Panomer's version of events, Alips 'was as if completely out of her good sense and memory because she saw that they wanted to take away their said goods'.[8] Thus, her decision to round up the locals to help her prevent these two strangers from stealing from her was not premeditated, but was the result of a temporary insanity brought on by her fear of the loss of their property.

In choosing to claim that Alips was mad, Robert le Panomer's letter drew on a wider understanding of the depredations of war as a potential catalyst for mental distress.[9] These letters were the despairing cry of a population affected by wars they were unable to avoid. The period under study includes some of the most serious fighting of the Hundred Years War in France, and letters about peasants who, according to their families, were driven mad by the destruction of their livelihood at the hands of the soldiers indicate that war was viewed as a traumatic event for the population at large. The French countryside provided

7 AN JJ 173 fo 22v no 44: 'parlans langage estrange que on ne entendoit point et ne savoit ou se cestoient bretons anglois escocoys ou autres gens'.

8 AN JJ 173 fo 22v no 44: 'fut comme toute hors de son bon sens et memoire pour ce quelle veoit quilz vouloient emport leurs diz biens'.

9 For more on these cases, see Pfau 2013b.

provisions for the armies that moved through their lands, whether those provisions were sought under the guise of payment for protection or as more direct looting. France was often in a state of turmoil and, in the imaginations of the general public, the pillaging and brigandage surrounding the war with England and the civil wars among the French nobility was detrimental to the livelihoods as well as to the mental stability of the people.[10]

Letters mentioning madness as a result of pillaging appeared most regularly during the period of English rule and civil war,[11] and most were written to explain suicides. In the summer months of 1424, in fact, three different women were granted remission for committing suicide because of madness brought on by the wars being fought in their neighborhood. Although some men committed suicide due to losses caused by war, in

10 It is clearly beyond the scope of this study to enter into the continuing debate over whether the French peasants were the greatest sufferers in the Hundred Years War, and whether their sufferings contributed to the peasant uprisings of the period, but it is worth noting the ways remission letters have been used in support of this argument and what that means for any reading of these particular narratives. Jules Michelet's *Histoire de France* was the first book to posit the thesis, and there have been many other proponents and opponents since. Michelet 1876, vol. 4, p. 287: 'Les souffrances du paysan avaient passé la mesure; tous avaient frappé dessus, comme une bête tombée sous la charge; la bête se releva enragée, et elle mordit [...]. Dans cette guerre chevaleresque que se faisaient à armes courtoises les nobles de France et d'Angleterre, il n'y avait au fond qu'un ennemi, une victime des maux de la guerre; c'était le paysan'. Christopher Allmand has carried on Michelet's argument, although he focuses on peasant suffering, making use of the term 'non-combatants' to refer to the fourteenth- and fifteenth-century peasants, and relying on sermon literature and supplications to the papal court by French churches to show that these peasants' livelihoods were affected by the war. Allmand first proposed this terminology, which he took from contemporary discussion of the Vietnam War, in Allmand 1971, but it can also be found in Allmand 1988 and Allmand 1999. Nicholas Wright, though he does not deny that peasants did indeed suffer, insists the combatants suffered as well. He notes that the wholesale destruction of peasant property would not have been in the best interest of the nobility, which depended on peasant land cultivation for food, and points out the acknowledged differences between the noble armies and the brigands and pillagers who took advantage of the war to wreak havoc in the countryside. He also suggests that the peasants were willing and able to fight back, using remission letters as evidence of brigandage and peasant resistance. See Wright 1983a; Wright 1998; Wright 1983b; and Wright 1991.

11 France's political situation was particularly messy during and after Charles VI's reign. Through the Treaty of Troyes, arranged in 1420, Charles VI disinherited his son, Charles, in favor of the English king, Henry V, who married Charles VI's daughter Catherine. Henry V became regent of France until Charles VI's death, but Henry died in 1422, mere months before Charles, who left his newborn grandson, Henry VI of England, as king of France. Charles VII set himself up as an alternative monarch in the Loire valley, but was unable to retake Paris and the north until Joan of Arc came to his aid in 1429. Indeed, even with her help, it was not until 1438 that Charles VII finally replaced the English rule. For more on all of this, see Allmand 1988; Autrand 1986; Famiglietti 1986; and Guenée 2004.

these cases madness was not mentioned as an ancillary reason.[12] While suicide does not seem to have been considered a gendered response to war, madness leading to suicide appears to have been.[13] Indeed, the only references to the madness of men related to war was to the 'youthful folly' of those men seeking remission for fighting for the 'enemy' or becoming a brigand, and the 'lack of sense' that caused a man who had lost his livelihood during the war to violate trade sanctions by selling food to the enemy, or in enemy-occupied territory.[14]

One war-related case appeared in a letter from May of 1424, when Henriette, wife of Jehan Charnel, committed suicide in the town of Montagny-Sainte-Félicité near Senlis. According to her family and relatives, a company of soldiers had come to Montagny looking for provisions while Jehan Charnel was away in Picardy selling apples. The soldiers found Jehan Charnel's mare and appropriated it and two robes from Charnel's house. Henriette attempted to prevent them, but was so badly beaten for her pains that she lay bedridden for fifteen days afterwards. Eight days later, the soldiers returned and found their second horse. This time Jehan Charnel, who had returned home, tried to prevent them, but he was no more successful than his wife. When the bedridden Henriette was told that their second horse was gone, as well, she was so angered and displeased that she became 'troubled in her good sense and memory', saying several times each day that they had lost everything by losing their horses.[15] This narrative suggested that Henriette's anger at losing everything provided sufficient cause for her to go out of her mind and hang herself. The idea that the loss of goods could lead to madness appears in several letters. Perrote de Courcelles, another woman who went mad due to the depredations of war had, according to the letter composed by her family and relatives, 'lost her family and goods such that from anger and displeasure about it she was made to fall into a

12 See AN JJ 130 fo 152v no 269 (in 1387) and AN JJ 166 fo 213 no 317 (in 1412).

13 Despite the concentration on the tangible negative effects of war on peasants in the French countryside, none of the many articles and books on the topic have considered psychological aspects. One recent study on women's roles during the Hundred Years War uses chronicle accounts and some letters to valorize the women in question, without addressing the ways in which these narratives of strong women or of entire communities, including women, joining in to help with the defense of a town may reflect the desires and goals of the chronicler or letter-writer. See Gilbert 2005.

14 For the 'folie et jeunesse' leading to joining the enemy's army or brigandage, see AN JJ 172 fo 66 no 131 (in 1422); AN JJ 174 fo 101 no 228 (in 1428). For the 'non sens' or 'folie et ignorance' that caused people to sell flour or other foods to the enemy or in enemy-occupied lands, see AN JJ 172 fo 261 no 465 (in 1424); AN JJ 172 fo 310 no 558 (in 1423); and AN JJ 175 fo 133 no 369 (in 1434).

15 AN JJ 172 fo 266 no 474: 'troublee en son bon sens et memoire'.

sickness which held her for the space of four or five months from which she was totally idiotic without having true understanding'.[16] Here the loss described included not only goods but also people, without whom Perrote fell into an illness that led her to become mad and finally use a knife to cut her own throat. Thus, remission letters demonstrate the psychological as well as the material devastation of war.

However, despite the wider understanding of warfare as a cause of mental distress, the version of the narrative agreed upon by Guillaume and Alips le Paumier, Robin Germain, and Jehan Germain departed from Robert le Panomer's in multiple ways, and particularly in their choice not to attribute Alips' behavior to madness. The supplicants declared that they 'had no memory' of the exact date, just that it was around Saint Martin's day and after the conquest of Caen by the English.[17] By declaring their uncertainty about the date, the composers of these three letters established the uncertain nature of memory. Despite four witnesses who were able to agree on the details to the extent that they presented their cases in almost identical ways, no one could recall the exact date on which these events took place. This reminder of the fragility of human memories, particularly after the passage of time, could have been an effort to legitimize their own version of events as opposed to Robert le Panomer's.

The composers of the new narrative of events, unlike Robert, did not choose to provide a list of possible languages the two men might have been speaking, instead stating it was 'English or another language'.[18] This version of events also avoided representing the two men with drawn swords during their early interactions with Guillaume and Alips le Paumier. Instead, their threatening actions were directed towards the couple's goods, which they gathered together and seemed to plan to carry away. Indeed, it was because they could not understand these strangers, not because the strangers threatened them with bodily harm, that Guillaume and Alips became frightened and angry. According to their letter, Guillaume went to bed and Alips (without consulting her husband) left the house to complain to the neighbors about these two strangers. Significantly, these three letters did

16 AN JJ 172 fo 340 no 614: 'perdu ses amis et biens dont par courrouz et desplaisir de ce elle feust cheute en maladie laquelle la tenue par lespace de iiij a v mois dont elle estoit tout ediotte sans avoir vray entendement'.

17 AN JJ 173 fo 88 no 170, AN JJ 173 fo 88v no 171, and AN JJ 173 fo 89v no 172: 'dont lesdis suppliant ne sont recors'.

18 AN JJ 173 fo 88 no 170; AN JJ 173 fo 88v no 171; and AN JJ 173 fo 89v no 172: 'parlans anglois ou autre langage'.

not mention temporary madness as a mitigating factor for Alips's actions.[19] Madness could be a complicated claim to make, since it could lead to a mandate in the letter of remission forcing the family to keep the mad person locked up or under guard.[20] This was particularly true in Normandy where the law codes called for the restraint of the mad to prevent them from causing fires.[21] Clearly, Robert le Panomer did not find it problematic to refer to the temporary madness of his neighbor who called for his aid, whereas Guillaume and Alips le Paumier were hesitant to ascribe her behavior to madness. Instead, they presented her call for help as an understandable response to the threat of theft that the two strangers represented.

Robert le Panomer, the Paumiers, and the Germains were caught in an awkward moment of transition between political rivals, where alliances shifted and enemies became putative friends. On the ground, in local villages, these shifts engendered confusion, anger, and fear. Caen had fallen to the English forces, but residents of small towns in the countryside could not know in that moment how changes in policies at the level of kings and princes would color their own actions, reframing them in unexpected ways. From their perspective they had banded together as neighbors to defend their community from strangers with whom they were unable to communicate. Within three years, those strangers had, through the Treaty of Troyes, become allies. Within five years, the kingdoms of France and England were joined under a single king. As the first remission seeker, Robert le Panomer sought to emphasize the fear and confusion brought on by the unexplained actions of these two strangers, explaining that the men had drawn their swords and beaten the Palmiers. He described Alips le Paumier as out of her senses in an attempt to recapture the emotional tenor of the moment and explain why her neighbors were so quick to come to her aid. The later letters were more balanced in their portrayal of the two strangers and in their depiction of Alips's actions.

This book has sought to explore the multiple levels on which medieval conceptions of madness interacted with constructions of kinship and community. The madness of ordinary people was imagined as a threat to the community as a result of their inability to understand basic human interactions, and sometimes because of their unintended violent actions

19 AN JJ 173 fo 88 no 170; AN JJ 173 fo 88v no 171; and AN JJ 173 fo 89 no 172.

20 For example, the letter for Jehan de Moustier in AN JJ 114 fo 106v no 212 (in 1378) and one for Jehannecte Troppé in AN JJ 173 fo 33v no 63 (in 1425). Edited in Le Cacheux 1907–1908, vol. 1, pp. 181–183.

21 Gruchy 1881, p. 184.

against themselves or others. Nevertheless, the narratives written around these figures sought to reconstruct the kin and communal ties fractured by these mad people, reimagining local communities. Communities are constantly in the process of construction through the creation of boundaries and the affirmation of ties. Rather than being expelled, the mad were integrated, often through the use of surveillance or chains, into the bosom of their kin and communal relationships. Nevertheless, the use of the language of madness in these letters points to the instability of the very systems remission narratives sought to uphold.

Bibliography

Unpublished Primary Sources

Archives Nationales Series JJ books 78–229.
British Library Additional 11612.
British Library Egerton 737.
British Library Harley 4114.
British Library Lansdowne 1175.

Published Primary Sources

Albertanus of Brescia. 1873. 'Albertani Brixiensis Liber Consolationis et Consilii, ex quo hausta est fabula gallica de Melibeo et Prudentia, quam, anglice redditam et "The Tale of Melibe" inscriptam, Galfridus Chaucer inter "Canterbury Tales" recepit'. In, ed. Thor Sundby. N. Trübner & Co, http://freespace.virgin.net/angus.graham/Albertano.htm. Accessed 5/8/2007, 2007.

Aquinas, Thomas. 1964. *Summa Theologiae*. Edited by James J. Cunningham. 60 vols. London: Blackfriars.

———. 1981. *Summa Theologica*. Translated by Fathers of the English Dominican Province. 5 vols. Westminster, MD: Christian Classics.

Augustine. 1957. *The City of God against the Pagans*. Edited and translated by George E. McCracken. 7 vols. Cambridge, MA: Harvard University Press.

Beautemps-Beaupré, J., ed. 1883. *Coutumes et institutions de l'Anjou et du Maine antérieures au XVIe siècle*. 8 vols. Paris: Auguste Durand et Pedone-Lauriel.

Behrends, Okko, Rolf Knütel, and Theodor Mommsen, eds. 1995. *Corpus Iuris Civilis: Text und Übersetzung*. 3 vols. Heidelberg: C.F. Müller.

Bellaguet, M. L., ed. 1842. Reprint 1994. *Chronique du religieux de Saint-Denys contenant le règne de Charles VI de 1380 à 1422*. 6 vols., *Éditions du Comité des travaux historiques et scientifiques*. Paris: L'imprimerie de Crapelet.

Boccaccio, Giovanni. 1962. *De Casibus Illustrium Virorum: A Facsimile Reproduction of the Paris Edition of 1520*. Gainesville: Scholars' Facsimiles and Reprints.

Bonnardot, François, ed. 1884. *Le Psautier de Metz: Texte du xive siècle*. Paris: F. Vieweg.

Boyle, Brian, Andrew Byler, and Paul Halsall. 1996. 'Medieval Sourcebook: Mass of the Roman Rite'. In Paul Halsall, ed. https://sourcebooks.fordham.edu/basis/latinmass2.asp. Accessed 7/6/20, 2020.

Brant, Sebastian. 1962. *The Ship of Fools*. Edited and translated by Edwin H. Zeydel. New York: Dover Publications.

Challoner, Richard, ed. 1971. *The Holy Bible, Translated from the Latin Vulgate; Diligently Compared with the Hebrew, Greek, and other Editions in Divers Languages. The Old Testament First Published by the English College at Douay, A.D. 1609, and the New Testament First Published by the English College at Rheims, A.D. 1582.* Rockford, IL: Tan Books and Publishers.

Champion, Pierre, ed. 1920–1921. *Procès de condamnation de Jeanne d'Arc. Texte, traduction et notes.* 2 vols. Paris: E. Champion.

Chaplais, Pierre. 1982. *English Medieval Diplomatic Practice, Part I: Documents and Interpretation.* 2 vols. London: Her Majesty's Stationery Office.

Chevalier, Bernard, ed. 1993. *Les Pays de la Loire Moyenne dans le Trésor des Chartes: Berry, Blésois, Chartrain, Orléanais, Touraine 1350-1502 (Archives nationales, JJ 80–235) Collection de documents inédits sur l'histoire de France.* Paris: Comité des travaux historiques et scientifiques.

Chrétien de Troyes. 1994. *Le Chevalier au Lion; ou le Roman d'Yvain: Édition critique d'après le manuscrit B.N. fr. 1433.* Edited and translated by David F. Hult. Paris: Librairie Générale Française.

Dossat, Yves, Anne-Marie LeMason, and Philippe Wolff, eds. 1983. *Le Languedoc et le Rouergue dans le Trésor des Chartes.* Paris: Comité des travaux historiques et scientifiques.

Euripides. 2001. *The Bacchae.* Translated by Herbert Golder. New York: Applause Theatre & Cinema Books.

Fabri, Felix. 1896. *The Book of the Wanderings of Felix Fabri (Circa 1480-1483 A.D.).* Edited and translated by Aubrey Stewart. 2 vols. London: Palestine Pilgrims' Text Society.

Gathercole, Patricia May, ed. 1968. *Laurent de Premierfait's Des cas des nobles hommes et femmes, book 1, translated from Boccaccio, Studies in the Romance languages and literatures no. 74.* Chapel Hill: University of North Carolina Press.

Gerson, Jean. 1962. *Oeuvres complètes.* Edited by Mgr. Glorieux. 10 vols. Paris: Desclée & Cie.

———. 1998. 'On Distinguishing True from False Revelations'. In *Jean Gerson: Early Works*, edited by Brian Patrick McGuire, 334–364. New York: Paulist Press.

Gruchy, William Lawrence de, ed. 1881. *L'ancienne coutume de Normandie.* Jersey: C. LeFeuvre.

Guérin, Paul, ed. 1909. *Recueil des documents concernant le Poitou contenus dans les registres de la chancellerie de France, Archives historiques du Poitou.* 12 vols. Poitiers: Société française d'imprimerie et de librairie.

Guillaume de Lorris and Jean de Meun. 1992. *Le Roman de la Rose: Édition d'après les manuscrits BN 12786 et BN 378*. Edited by Armand Strubel. Paris: Librairie Générale Française.

Gut, Christian, ed. 1996. *Les pays de l'Oise sous la domination anglaise (1420-1435) d'après les registres de la Chancellerie de France*. Paris: Comité des travaux historiques et scientifiques.

Hansen, Bert. 1985. *Nicole Oresme and the Marvels of Nature: A Study of his De causis mirabilium with Critical Edition, Translation, and Commentary*. Toronto: Pontifical Institute of Mediaeval Studies.

Hobbins, Daniel. 2005. *The Trial of Joan of Arc*. Boston: Harvard University Press.

Institoris, Henricus, and Jacobus Sprenger. 2006. *Malleus Maleficarum*. Edited and translated by Christopher Mackay. 2 vols. Cambridge: Cambridge University Press.

Isidore of Seville. 1911. *Etymologies*. Edited by W. M. Lindsay. Oxford: Oxford University Press.

———. 2006. *The Etymologies of Isidore of Seville*. Translated by Stephen A. Barney, W. J. Lewis, J. A. Beach, and Oliver Berghof. Cambridge: Cambridge University Press.

Jacobus de Voragine. 1993. *The Golden Legend: Readings on the Saints*. Translated by William Granger Ryan. 2 vols. Princeton: Princeton University Press.

Jacques d' Ableiges. 1868. *Le grand coutumier de France*. Edited by Rodolphe Dareste and Édouard Laboulaye. Paris: Auguste Durand.

Jassemin, Henri-Frédéric, and Aline Vallée, eds. 1999. *Registres du Trésor des Chartes*. 3 vols. Vol. 2: Règnes des fils de Philippe le Bel, deuxième partie: règne de Charles IV le Bel. Paris: Imprimerie nationale.

Le Cacheux, Paul, ed. 1907–1908. *Actes de la chancellerie d'Henri VI concernant la Normandie sous la domination anglaise (1422–1435), extraits des registres du Trésor des chartes aux Archives nationales*. 2 vols. Rouen: A. Lestringant.

Longnon, Auguste, ed. 1878. *Paris pendant la domination anglaise (1420–1436): Documents extraits des registres de la Chancellerie de France*. Paris: H. Champion.

Maréchal, Michel, and Jacques Poumarède, eds. 1988. *La coutume de Saint-Sever (1380–1480): Édition et commentaire des textes gascon et latin*. Paris: Éditions du C.T.H.S.

McWebb, Christine, ed. 2006. *Debating the Roman de la Rose: A Critical Anthology*. London: Routledge.

Mommsen, Theodor, Paul Krueger, and Alan Watson, eds. 1985. *The Digest of Justinian*. 4 vols. Philadelphia: University of Pennsylvania Press.

Nider, Jean. 1999. 'Formicarius Livre II, chapitre 4, et Livre V, chapitre 3, 4, 7'. Edited by Catherine Chène. In *L'imaginaire du sabbat: Édition dritique des textes les plus anciens (1430 c. –1440 c.)*, edited by Martine Ostorero, Agostino Paravicini

Bagliani and Kathrin Utz Tremp. Lausanne: Section d'histoire, Faculté des lettres, Université de Lausanne.

Ovid. *Metamorphoses*. 2004. Translated by Charles Martin. New York: W.W. Norton.

Petit-Dutaillis, Charles Edmond, ed. 1908. *Documents nouveaux sur les mœurs populaires et le droit de vengeance dans les Pays-Bas au XVe siècle*. Paris: H. Champion.

Philippe de Beaumanoir. 1970–1974. *Coutumes de Beauvaisis*. Edited by Amédée Salmon. 3 vols. Paris: A. Picard et Fils.

———. 1992. *The Coutumes de Beauvaisis of Philippe de Beaumanoir*. Edited and translated by F.R.P. Akehurst. Philadelphia: University of Pennsylvania Press.

Pierre de Fenin. 1837. *Mémoires de Pierre de Fenin, comprenant le récit des événements qui se sont passés en France et en Bourgogne sous les règnes de Charles VI et Charles VII: 1407–1427*. Edited by L.M.E. Dupont, *Société de l'histoire de France*. Paris: J. Renouard.

Rapetti, Louis Nicolas, ed. 1850. *Li Livres de jostice et de plet, publié pour la première fois d'après le manuscrit unique de la Bibliothèque nationale, Collection de documents inédits sur l'histoire de France, 1. sér. Histoire politique*. Paris: Typographie de Firmin Didot frères.

Samaran, Charles, ed. 1966. *La Gascogne dans les registres du Trésor des Chartes Collection de documents inédits sur l'histoire de France*. Paris: Bibliothèque nationale.

Tanon, Louis, ed. 1877. *Registre criminel de la justice de St. Martin des Champs à Paris au XIVe siècle*. Paris: L. Willem.

Tardif, Ernest-Joseph, ed. 1903. *Coutumiers de Normandie: Textes critiques*. 2 vols. Vol. 1, *Le très ancien coutumier de Normandie* Paris: A. Picard et Fils.

Vilevault, Louis-Guillaume de, and Louis George Oudard-Feudrix de Bréquigny, eds. 1763. *Ordonnances des Rois de France de la 3e Race: Dixième volume, Contenant les ordonnances de Charles VI, données depuis le commencement de l'année 1411 jusqu'à la fin de l'année 1418*. 22 vols. Paris: Imprimerie royale.

Weber, Robert, ed. 1969. Reprint 1994. *Biblia Sacra Iuxta Vulgatam Versionem*. Stuttgart: Deutsche Bibelgesellschaft.

Secondary Sources

Akehurst, F.R.P. 2003. 'Good Name, Reputation, and Notoriety in French Customary Law'. In *Fama: The Politics of Talk and Reputation in Medieval Europe*, edited by Thelma Fenster and Daniel Lord Smail, 75–94. Ithaca: Cornell University Press.

Allmand, Christopher. 1971. 'The War and the Non-combatant'. In *The Hundred Years War*, edited by Kenneth Fowler, 163–183. London: MacMillan Press.

———. 1988. *The Hundred Years War: England and France at War c. 1300–c.1450*. Cambridge: Cambridge University Press.

———. 1999. 'War and the Non-Combatant in the Middle Ages'. In *Medieval Warfare: A History*, edited by Maurice Keen, 253–272. Oxford: Oxford University Press.

Anderson, Benedict. 1983. *Imagined Communities: Reflections on the Origin and Spread of Nationalism*. London: Verso.

Andrews, Jonathan, and Andrew Scull. 2003. *Customers and Patrons of the Mad-trade: The Management of Lunacy in Eighteenth-century London*. Berkeley: University of California Press.

Arnade, Peter and Walter Prevenier. 2015. *Honor, Vengeance, and Social Trouble: Pardon Letters in the Burgundian Low Countries*. Ithaca: Cornell University Press.

Arnold, John H. 2001. *Inquisition and Power: Catharism and the Confessing Subject in Medieval Languedoc*. Philadelphia: University of Pennsylvania Press.

Autrand, Françoise. 1986. *Charles VI: La folie du roi*. Paris: Fayard.

Babbitt, Susan M. 1985. 'Oresme's *Livre de Politiques* and the France of Charles V'. *Transactions of the American Philosophical Society, New Series* 75, no. 1: 1–158.

Backman, E. Louis. 1977. *Religious Dances in the Christian Church and in Popular Medicine*. Translated by E. Classen. Westport, CT: Greenwood Press.

Barasch, Moshe. 1999. 'Despair in the Medieval Imagination'. *Social Research* 66, no. 2: 565–576.

Beattie, Cordelia. 2006. 'Single Women, Work, and Family: The Chancery Dispute of Jane Wynde and Margaret Clerk'. In *Voices from the Bench: The Narratives of Lesser Folk in Medieval Trials*, edited by Michael Goodich, 177–202. New York: Palgrave Macmillan.

Bell, Rudolph M. 1985. *Holy Anorexia*. Chicago: University of Chicago Press.

Beresford, Peter. 2000. 'What Have Madness and Psychiatric System Survivors Got to Do with Disability and Disability Studies?' *Disability and Society* 15, no. 1:167–172.

———. 2019. '"Mad", Mad Studies and Advancing Inclusive Resistance'. *Disability and Society*: https://doi.org/10.1080/09687599.2019.1692168 Accessed 5/11/20, 2020.

Berger, Samuel. 1884. Reprint 1967. *La Bible française au moyen âge*. Paris: Imprimerie nationale. Reprint, Genève, Slatkine Reprints.

Bernheimer, Richard. 1952. *Wild Men in the Middle Ages: A Study in Art, Sentiment, and Demonology*. Cambridge, MA: Harvard University Press.

Biddick, Kathleen. 1989. *The Other Economy: Pastoral Husbandry on a Medieval Estate*. Berkeley: University of California Press.

Bloch, Marc. 1967. *Land and Work in Mediaeval Europe*. Translated by J. E. Anderson. New York: Routledge.

Boswell, John. 1988. *The Kindness of Strangers: The Abandonment of Children in Western Europe from Late Antiquity to the Renaissance*. New York: Pantheon Books.

Bozzolo, Carla, ed. 2004. *Un traducteur et un humaniste de l'époque de Charles V: Laurent de Premierfait*. Paris: Publications de la Sorbonne.

Briggs, Robin. 1989. *Communities of Belief: Cultural and Social Tension in Early Modern France*. Oxford: Clarendon Press.

———. 1996. *Witches and Neighbors: The Social and Cultural Context of European Witchcraft*. London: Harper Collins.

Brissaud, Y.-B. 1962. 'L'infanticide à la fin du moyen âge, ses motivations pyschologiques et sa répression'. *Revue historique de droit français et étrange* 50: 240–242.

———. 1971. 'Le droit de grâce à la fin du moyen-âge (XIVeme siècle – XVeme siècle): Contribution à l'étude de la restauration de la souveraineté monarchique.' PhD dissertation, Université de Poitiers.

Broedel, Hans Peter. 2003. *The Malleus Maleficarum and the Construction of Witchcraft: Theology and Popular Belief.* Manchester: Manchester University Press.

Brundage, James. 1987. *Law, Sex, and Christian Society in Medieval Europe*. Chicago: University of Chicago Press.

———. 1995. *Medieval Canon Law*. London: Longman.

———. 2004. *The Profession and Practice of Medieval Canon Law*. Aldershot, Hampshire: Ashgate.

Butler, Sara M. 2006. 'Degrees of Culpability: Suicide Verdicts, Mercy, and the Jury in Medieval England'. *Journal of Medieval and Early Modern Studies* 36, no. 2: 263–290.

———. 2015. *Forensic Medicine and Death Investigation in Medieval England*. New York: Routledge.

Bynum, Caroline Walker. 1984. 'Did the Twelfth Century Discover the Individual?' In *Jesus as Mother: Studies in the Spirituality of the High Middle Ages*, 82–109. Berkeley: University of California Press.

———. 1987. *Holy Feast and Holy Fast: The Religious Significance of Food to Medieval Women*. Berkeley: University of California Press.

Bynum, W.F., Roy Porter, and Michael Shepherd, eds. 1985. *The Anatomy of Madness: Essays in the History of Psychiatry*. 2 Vols. London: Tavistock Publications.

Caciola, Nancy. 2000. 'Mystics, Demoniacs, and the Physiology of Spirit Possession in Medieval Europe'. *Comparative Studies in Society and History* 42, no. 2: 268–306.

———. 2003. *Discerning Spirits: Divine and Demonic Possession in the Middle Ages*. Ithaca: Cornell University Press.

Canning, Kathleen. 2006. *Gender History in Practice: Historical Perspectives on Bodies, Class, and Citizenship*. Ithaca: Cornell University Press.

Chambers, David S., and Trevor Dean. 1997. *Clean Hands and Rough Justice: An Investigating Magistrate in Renaissance Italy*. Ann Arbor: University of Michigan Press.

Chène, Catherine. 1999. 'Introduction'. In *L'imaginaire du sabbat: Édition critique des textes les plus anciens (1430 c. – 1440 c.)*, edited by Martine Ostorero, Agostino Paravicini Bagliani, and Kathrin Utz Tremp, 101–120. Lausanne: Section d'histoire, Faculté des lettres, Université de Lausanne.

Clarke, Gillian. 1992. 'Town and Countryside in Medieval Italy: A Critical Evaluation of the Sources for Understanding the Mechanisms of Supply and Demand'. *Anthropozoologica* 16: 75–82.

Cohen, Esther. 1990. '"To Die a Criminal for the Public Good": The Execution Ritual in Late Medieval Paris'. In *Law, Custom, and the Social Fabric in Medieval Europe: Essays in Honor of Bryce Lyon*, edited by Bernard S. Bachrach and David Nicholas, 285–304. Kalamazoo, MI: Medieval Institute Publications.

———. 1993. *The Crossroads of Justice: Law and Culture in Late Medieval France*. New York: E.J. Brill.

Cohn, Norman. 1975. *Europe's Inner Demons: An Enquiry Inspired by the Great Witch-hunt*. London: Sussex University Press.

Combes, André. 1973. *Jean de Montreuil et le Chancelier Gerson: Contribution à l'histoire des rapports de l'humanisme et de la théologie en France au début du xve siècle*. Second ed., *Études de Philosophie Médiévale*. Paris: Librairie Philosophique J. Vrin.

Courtenay, William J. 2000. 'The Early Career of Nicole Oresme'. *Isis* 91, no. 3: 542–548.

Coville, Alfred. 1932. *Jean Petit: La question du tyrannicide au commencement du XVe siècle*. Paris: A. Picard.

———. 1934. *Gontier et Pierre Col et l'humanisme en France au temps de Charles VI*. Paris: Librairie E. Droz.

Crane, Susan. 2002. *The Performance of Self: Ritual, Clothing, and Identity during the Hundred Years War*. Philadelphia: University of Pennsylvania Press.

Davis, Natalie Zemon. 1981. 'The Possibilities of the Past: Anthropology and History'. *Journal of Interdisciplinary History* 12, no. 2, The New History: The 1980s and Beyond (II): 267–275.

———. 1987. *Fiction in the Archives: Pardon Tales and their Tellers in Sixteenth-century France*. Stanford, CA: Stanford University Press.

Dean, Trevor. 2001. *Crime in Medieval Europe: 1200–1500*. Harlow: Pearson Education Limited.

Deploige, Jeroen. 2005. 'Studying Emotions: The Medievalist as Human Scientist?' In *Emotions in the Heart of the City (14th – 16th century)*, edited by Elodie Lecuppre-Desjardin and Anne-Laure Van Bruaene, 3–24. Turnhout: Brepols.

Desjardins, Mireille. 1997. 'Les savoirs des notaires et secrétaires du roi et la géographie de la france d'après le manuel d'Odart Morchesne et un index de chancellerie'. In *Écrit et pouvoir dans les chancelleries médiévales: Espace français, espace anglais*, edited by Kouky Fianu and DeLloyd J. Guth, 87–97. Louvain-la-neuve: Collège Cardinal Mercier.

Doll, Monika. 2003. *Haustierhaltung und Schlachtsitten des Mittelalters und der Neuzeit: Ein Synthese aus Archäozoologischen, Bildlichen und Schriftlichen Quellen Mitteleuropas*. Rahden: Internationale Archäologie.

Doob, Penelope. 1974. *Nebuchadnezzar's Children: Conventions in Madness in Middle English Literature*. New Haven: Yale University Press.

Dunbabin, Jean. 2002. *Captivity and Imprisonment in Medieval Europe, 1000–1300*. Edited by Miri Rubin, *Medieval Culture and Society*. New York: Palgrave MacMillan.

Dunn, Maryjane, and Linda Davidson. 2000. 'Pilgrimage Sites, Spanish'. In *Trade, Travel, and Exploration in the Middle Ages: An Encyclopedia*, edited by John Block Friedman, Kristen Mossler Figg, Scott D. Westrem, and Gregory G. Guzman, 484–488. New York: Garland.

Elias, Norbert. 1978. *The Civilizing Process*. Translated by Edmund Jephcott. New York: Urizen Books.

Evans, G. R. 2002. *Law and Theology in the Middle Ages*. London: Routledge.

Evans, Richard J. 1999. *In Defense of History*. New York: W. W. Norton.

Famiglietti, R.C. 1986. *Royal Intrigue: Crisis at the Court of Charles VI, 1392–1420*. New York: AMS Press.

———. 2004. 'Laurent de Premierfait: The Career of a Humanist in Early Fifteenth-Century Paris'. In *Un traducteur et un humaniste de l'époque de Charles V: Laurent de Premierfait*, edited by Carla Bozzolo, 31–51. Paris: Publications de la Sorbonne.

Fassler, Margot. 2007. '*Adventus* at Chartres: Ritual Models for Major Processions'. In *Ceremonial Culture in Pre-modern Europe*, edited by Nicholas Howe, 13–62. Notre Dame: University of Notre Dame Press.

Finucane, Ronald C. 1977. *Miracles and Pilgrims: Popular Beliefs in Medieval England*. London: Dent.

Firnhaber-Baker, Justine. 2006. 'From God's Peace to the King's Order: Late Medieval Limitations on Non-Royal Warfare'. *Essays in Medieval Studies* 23: 19–30.

———. 2007. '"Guerram publice et palam faciendo": Local War and Royal Authority in Late Medieval Southern France'. PhD dissertation, Harvard University.

———. 2014. *Violence and the State in Languedoc, 1250–1400*. Cambridge: Cambridge University Press.

Flanigan, C. Clifford. 2001. 'The Moving Subject: Medieval Liturgical Processions in Semiotic and Cultural Perspective'. In *Moving Subjects: Processional Performance in the Middle Ages and Renaissance*, edited by Kathleen Ashley and Wim Hüsken, 35–52. Amsterdam: Rodopi B.V.

Forde, Simon, Lesley Johnson, and Alan V. Murray, eds. 1995. *Concepts of National Identity in the Middle Ages*. Leeds: University Printing Service at the University of Leeds.

Foucault, Michel. 1961. *Folie et Déraison. Histore de la folie à l'âge classique*. Paris: Plon.

———. 1965. *Madness and Civilization: A History of Insanity in the Age of Reason*. Translated by Richard Howard. New York: Random House.

———. 1972. *Histoire de la folie à l'âge classique. Suivi de Mon corps, ce papier, ce feu et La folie, l'absence d'œuvre*. Paris: Gallimard.

———. 2006. *History of Madness*. Translated by Jean Khalfa and Jonathan Murphy. London: Routledge.

François, Michel. 1942. 'Note sur les lettres de rémission transcrites dans les registres du Trésor des Chartes'. *Bibliothèque de l'École des Chartes* 103: 317–324.

Fritz, Jean-Marie. 1992. *Le discours du fou au Moyen Age: XIIe–XIIIe siècles*. Paris: Presses Universitaires de France.

Gauvard, Claude. 1991. *'De Grace Especial': Crime, état et société en France à la fin du Moyen Age*. 2 vols. Paris: Publications de la Sorbonne.

———. 1995. 'Grâce et exécution capitale: Les deux visages de la justice royale française à la fin du moyen âge'. In *La Justice Royale et le Parlement de Paris (XIVe–XVIIe siècle)* edited by Yves-Marie Bercé and Alfred Soman, 275–290. Paris: H. Champion.

———. 1997. 'Les clercs de la chancellerie royale française et l'écriture des lettres de rémission aux XIVe et XVe siècles'. In *Écrit et pouvoir dans les chancelleries médiévales: Espace français, espace anglais*, edited by Kouky Fianu and DeLloyd J. Guth, 281–292. Louvain-la-neuve: Collège Cardinal Mercier.

———. 1999. 'Fear of Crime in Late Medieval France'. In *Medieval Crime and Social Control*, edited by Barbara Hanawalt and David Wallace, 1–48. Minneapolis: University of Minnesota Press.

Gauvard, Claude, and Gilbert Ouy. 2001. 'Gerson et l'infanticide: Défense des femmes et critique de la pénitence publique'. In *'Riens ne m'est seur que la chose incertaine': Études sur l'art d'écrire au Moyen Âge offertes à Eric Hicks par ses élèves, collègues, amies et amis*, edited by Jean-Claude Mühlethaler, Denis Billotte, Alain Corbellari, Marie-Thérèse Bonadonna, and Barbara Wahlen, 45–66. Genève: Éditions Slatkine.

Geremek, Bronislaw. 1968. *Le salariat dans l'artisanat parisien aux XIIIe–XVe siècles; étude sur le marché de la main-d'oeuvre au Moyen Age*. Translated by Anna Posner and Christiane Klapisch-Zuber. Paris: Mouton.

Gilbert, James E. 2005. 'A Medieval "Rosie the Riveter"? Women in France and Southern England during the Hundred Years War'. In *Hundred Years War: A Wider Focus*, edited by L.J. Andrew Villalon and Donald J. Kagey, 333–361. Leiden: Brill.

Goffman, Erving. 1962. *Asylums: Essays on the Social Situation of Mental Patients and other Inmates*. Chicago: Aldine Pub. Co.

Gonthier, Nicole. 1992. *Cris de haine et rites d'unité: La violence dans les villes, XIIIe–XVIe siècle*. Turnhout: Brepols.

———. 1993. *Délinquance, justice et société dans le Lyonnais médieval: De la fin du XIIIe siècle au début du XVIe siècle*. Paris: Éditions Arguments.

———. 1998. *Le châtiment du crime au Moyen Âge*. Rennes: Presses Universitaires de Rennes.

Gordon, Colin. 1992. '*Histoire de la folie*: An Unknown Book by Michel Foucault'. In *Rewriting the History of Madness: Studies in Foucault's Histoire de la folie*, edited by Arthur Still and Irving Velody, 19–42. London: Routledge.

Gove, Walter. 1979. 'The Labeling Versus the Psychiatric Explanation of Mental Illness: A Debate That Has Become Substantively Irrelevant: Reply'. *Journal of Health and Social Behavior* 20, no. 3: 301–304.

Green, Thomas A. 1972. 'Societal Concepts of Criminal Liability for Homicide in Mediaeval England'. *Speculum* 47, no. 4: 669–694.

Groebner, Valentin. 2007. *Who Are You?: Identification, Deception, and Surveillance in Early Modern Europe*. Translated by Mark Kyburz and John Peck. New York: Zone Books.

Guenée, Bernard. 1999. 'Liturgie et Politique: Les processions spéciales à Paris sous Charles VI'. In *Saint-Denis et la Royauté: Études Offertes à Bernard Guenée*, edited by Françoise Autrand, Claude Gauvard, and Jean-Marie Moeglin, 23–49. Paris: Publications de la Sorbonne.

———. 2004. *La folie de Charles VI: Roi Bien-Aimé*. Paris: Perrin.

———, and Françoise Lehoux. 1968. *Les entrées royales françaises de 1328 à 1515*. Paris: Éditions du Centre national de la recherche scientifique.

Gut, Christian. 2000. 'Autour des registres de la chancellerie française de Henri VI, roi de France et d'Angleterre'. In *Pouvoir, Justice et Société*, edited by Jacqueline Hoareau-Dodinau and Pascal Texier, 81–99. Limoges: Presses universitaires de Limoges.

Hanawalt, Barbara. 1974. 'The Peasant Family and Crime in Fourteenth-Century England'. *The Journal of British Studies* 13, no. 2: 1–18.

———. 1979. *Crime and Conflict in English Communities, 1300–1348*. Cambridge, MA: Harvard University Press.

———. 1986. *The Ties that Bound: Peasant Families in Medieval England*. Oxford: Oxford University Press.

———. 1998. *'Of Good and Ill Repute': Gender and Social Control in Medieval England*. New York: Oxford University Press.

Harper, Stephen. 2003. *Insanity, Individuals, and Society in Late-Medieval English Literature: The Subject of Madness*. Lewiston: Edwin Mellen Press.

Harvey, E. Ruth. 1975. *The Inward Wits: Psychological Theory in the Middle Ages and the Renaissance* London: Warburg Institute, University of London.

Heers, Jacques. 1977. *Family Clans in the Middle Ages: A Study of Political and Social Structures in Urban Areas*. Translated by Barry Herbert. Amsterdam: North-Holland Publishing Company.

Henisch, Bridget Ann. 1999. *The Medieval Calendar Year*. University Park: Pennsylvania State University Press.

Herlihy, David. 1983. 'The Making of the Medieval Family: Symmetry, Structure, and Sentiment'. *Journal of Family History* 8, no. 2: 116–130.

———. 1985. *Medieval Households*. Cambridge, MA: Harvard University Press.

Herlihy, David, and Christiane Klapisch-Zuber. 1985. *Tuscans and their Families: A Study of the Florentine Catasto of 1427*. New Haven: Yale University Press.

Hoareau-Dodinau, Jacqueline. 1999. 'La jeune fille, le roi et le pendu: À propos de la grâce par mariage'. In *Le Pardon*, edited by Jacqueline Hoareau-Dodinau, Xavier Rousseaux, and Pascal Texier, 353–372. Limoges: Presses universitaires de Limoges.

———. 2001. 'L'animal devant son juge: Coupable ou victime?' In *La culpabilité: Actes des XXèmes Journées d'histoire du droit, Limoges*, edited by Jacqueline Hoareau-Dodinau and Pascal Texier, 187–201. Limoges: Presses universitaires de Limoges.

———. 2002. *Dieu et le roi: La répression du blasphème et de l'injure au roi à la fin du moyen âge*. Limoges: Presses universitaires de Limoges.

Holbrook, Sue Ellen. 2006. 'The Properties of Things and Textual Power: Illustrating the French Translation of *De Proprietatibus Rerum* and a Latin Precursor'. In *Patrons, Authors, and Workshops: Books and Book Production in Paris around 1400*, edited by Godfried Croenen and Peter Ainsworth, 367–404. Louvain: Peeters.

Hughes, Diane Owen. 1975. 'Domestic Ideals and Social Behavior: Evidence from Medieval Genoa'. In *The Family in History*, edited by Charles E. Rosenberg, 115–143. Philadelphia: University of Pennsylvania Press.

———. 2004. 'Bodies, Disease and Society'. In *Italy in the Age of the Renaissance*, edited by John M. Najemy, 103–123. Oxford: Oxford University Press.

Huizinga, Johan. 1954. *The Waning of the Middle Ages: A Study of the Forms of Life, Thought and Art in France and the Netherlands in the XIVth and XVth Centuries*. Garden City, NY: Doubleday and Company.

Huot, Sylvia. 1993. *The Romance of the Rose and its Medieval Readers: Interpretation, Reception, Manuscript Transmission*. Cambridge: Cambridge University Press.

———. 2003. *Madness in Medieval French Literature: Identities Found and Lost*. Oxford: Oxford University Press.

Jacquart, Danielle. 1980. 'Le regard d'un médecin sur son temps: Jacques Despars (1380?-1458)'. *Bibliothèque de l'Ecole des chartes 138*, 35–86. Paris-Genève: Librairie Droz.

———. 2001. 'Moses, Galen and Jacques Despars: Religious Orthodoxy as a Path to Unorthodox Medical Views'. In *Religion and Medicine in the Middle Ages,* edited by Peter Biller and Joseph Ziegler, 33–46. Woodbridge, Suffolk: Boydell and Brewer.

Jaeger, C. Stephen. 1985. *The Origins of Courtliness: Civilizing Trends and the Formation of Courtly Ideals, 939–1210*. Philadelphia: University of Pennsylvania Press.

Johnston, David. 1999. *Roman Law in Context.* Cambridge: Cambridge University Press.

Jolly, Karen, Catharina Raudvere, and Edward Peters. 2002. *Witchcraft and Magic in Europe Volume 3: The Middle Ages*. 6 vols. Edited by Bengt Ankarloo and Stuart Clark. Philadelphia: University of Pennsylvania Press.

Karlsen, Carol. 1987. *The Devil in the Shape of a Woman: Witchcraft in Colonial New England.* New York: Norton.

Klapisch-Zuber, Christiane. 1985. 'Blood Parents and Milk Parents: Wet Nursing in Florence, 1300-1500'. In *Women, Family, and Ritual in Renaissance Italy*, 132–164. Chicago: University of Chicago Press.

Klibansky, Raymond, Erwin Panofsky, and Fritz Saxl. 1964. *Saturn and Melancholoy: Studies in the History of Natural Philosophy, Religion, and Art.* London: Nelson.

Koenig, Anne M. 2020. 'Shipping Fools: Foucault's Wandering Madman and Civic Responsibility in Late Medieval Germany', *Journal of Social History* 54, no. 1: 1–36.

Kuehn, Thomas. 2003. '*Fama* as a Legal Status in Renaissance Florence'. In *Fama: The Politics of Talk and Reputation in Medieval Europe*, edited by Thelma Fenster and Daniel Lord Smail, 27–46. Ithaca: Cornell University Press.

Kuttner, Stephan. 1935. *Kanonistische Schuldlehre von Gratian bis auf die Dekretalen Gregors IX.* Vatican City: Biblioteca Apostolica Vaticana.

Ladurie, Emmanuel LeRoy. 1978. *Montaillou: The Promised Land of Error.* Translated by Barbara Bray. New York: Random House.

Laharie, Muriel. 1991. *La Folie au Moyen Âge: XIe–XIIIe siècles.* Paris: Le Léopard d'Or.

Lapeyre, André, and Rémy Scheurer. 1978. *Les notaires et secrétaires du roi sous les règnes de Louis XI, Charles VIII et Louis XII (1461–1515)*. 2 vols. Paris: Bibliothèque Nationale.

Laskaris, Julie. 2002. *The Art is Long: On the Sacred Disease and the Scientific Tradition.* Leiden: Brill.

Leeuwen, Jacqueline Van. 2005. 'Emotions on Trial: Attitudes towards the Sensitivity of Victims and Judges in Medieval Flanders'. In *Emotions in the Heart of the City (14th–16th centuries)* edited by Elodie Lecuppre-Desjardin and Anne-Laure Van Bruaene, 157–175. Turnhout: Brepols.

Lewis, P.S. 1965. 'War Propaganda and Historiography in Fifteenth-Century France and England'. *Transactions of the American Philosophical Society, 5th Series* 15: 1–21.

MacDonald, Michael. 1981. *Mystical Bedlam: Madness, Anxiety, and Healing in Seventeenth-century England*. Cambridge: Cambridge University Press.

Mansfield, Mary. 1995. *The Humiliation of Sinners: Public Penance in Thirteenth-Century France*. Ithaca: Cornell University Press.

Maxwell-Stuart, P.G. 2007. 'Introduction'. In *The Malleus Maleficarum*, edited by P.G. Maxwell-Stuart. Manchester: Manchester University Press.

Maza, Sarah C. 1993. *Private Lives and Public Affairs: The Causes Célèbres of Pre-revolutionary France*. Berkeley: University of California Press.

McCleery, Iona. 2005. 'Saintly Physician, Diabolical Doctor, Medieval Saint: Exploring the Reputation of Gil de Santarem in Medieval and Renaissance Portugal'. *Portuguese Studies* 21: 112–125.

McDonough, Susan Alice. 2013. *Witnesses, Neighbors, and Community in Late Medieval Marseille*. New York: Palgrave Macmillan.

Mellyn, Elizabeth W. 2014. *Mad Tuscans and Their Families: A History of Mental Disorder in Early Modern Italy*. Philadelphia: University of Pennsylvania Press.

Metzler, Irina. 2006. *Disability in Medieval Europe: Thinking about Physical Impairment during the High Middle Ages, c. 1100–1400*. London: Routledge.

———. 2016. *Fools and idiots? Intellectual disability in the Middle Ages*. Manchester: Manchester University Press.

Meyerson, Mark D. 2004. 'The Murder of Pau de Saint Martí: Jews, *Conversos*, and the Feud in Fifteenth-Century Valencia'. In *'A Great Effusion of Blood'? Interpreting Medieval Violence*, edited by Mark D. Meyerson, Daniel Thiery, and Oren Falk. Toronto: University of Toronto Press.

Michelet, Jules. 1876. *Histoire de France: Nouvelle édition, revue et augmentée*. 19 vols. Paris: Librairie Abel Pilon.

Midelfort, H.C. Erik. 1980. 'Madness and Civilization in Early Modern Europe: A Reappraisal of Michel Foucault'. In *After the Reformation: Essays in Honor of J.H. Hexter*, edited by Barbara Malament, 247–265. Philadelphia: University of Pennsylvania Press.

———. 1994. *Mad Princes of Renaissance Germany*. Charlottesville: University of Virginia Press.

———. 1999. *A History of Madness in Sixteenth-Century Germany*. Stanford: Stanford University Press.

Mink, Louis O. 1981. 'Everyman His or Her own Annalist'. *Critical Inquiry* 7, no. 4: 777–783.

Mollat, Michel. 1986. *The Poor in the Middle Ages: An Essay in Social History*. Translated by Arthur Goldhammer. New Haven: Yale University Press.

Moore, R. I. 1987. *The Formation of a Persecuting Society: Power and Deviance in Western Europe, 950–1250*. Oxford: Blackwell.

Mortimer, Nigel. 2005. *John Lydgate's Fall of Princes: Narrative Tragedy in its Literary and Political Contexts*. Oxford: Clarendon Press.

Muchembled, Robert. 1989. *La Violence au village: Sociabilité et comportements populaires en Artois du XVe au XVIIe siècle*. Turnhout: Brepols.

Muir, Edward. 1993. *Mad Blood Stirring: Vendetta and Factions in Friuli during the Renaissance*. Baltimore: Johns Hopkins University Press.

Murray, Alexander. 1998. *Suicide in the Middle Ages, Volume I: The Violent against Themselves*. 2 vols. Oxford: Oxford University Press.

Nalle, Sara Tilghman. 2001. *Mad for God: Bartolomé Sánchez, the Secret Messiah of Cardenete*. Charlottesville: University of Virginia Press.

Neaman, Judith. 1975. *Suggestion of the Devil: The Origins of Madness*. New York: Anchor Books.

Neugebauer, Richard. 1996. 'Mental Handicap in Medieval and Early Modern England: Criteria, Measurement and Care'. In *From Idiocy to Mental Deficiency: Historical Perspectives on People with Learning Disabilities*, edited by David Wright and Anne Digby. London: Routledge.

Neveux, François. 1987. *L'évêque Pierre Cauchon*. Paris: Denoël.

Newman, Barbara. 1998. 'Possessed by the Spirit: Devout Women, Demoniacs, and the Apostolic Life in the Thirteenth Century'. *Speculum* 73, no. 3: 733–770.

Nirenberg, David. 1996. *Communities of Violence: Persecution of Minorities in the Middle Ages*. Princeton: Princeton University Press.

'Opération Charles VI'. Laboratoire de Médiévistique occidentale de Paris. https://www.vjf.cnrs.fr/charlesVI/accueil.php Accessed May 19, 2020.

Paravy, Pierrette. 1979. 'À propos de la genèse médiévale des chasses aux sorcières: Le traité de Claude Tholosan, juge dauphinois (vers 1436)'. *Mélanges de l'École française de Rome* 91: 333–379.

Park, Katharine. 1988. 'The Organic Soul'. In *The Cambridge History of Renaissance Philosophy*, edited by Charles B. Schmitt, Quentin Skinner, Eckhard Kessler, and Jill Kraye, 464–484. Cambridge: Cambridge University Press.

Parlopiano, Brandon. 2013. 'Madmen and Lawyers: The Development and Practices of the Jurisprudence of Insanity in the Middle Ages.' PhD Dissertation, The Catholic University of America.

Perler, Dominik, ed. 2001. *Ancient and Medieval Theories of Intentionality*. Leiden: Brill.

Peters, Edward. 1990. 'Wounded Names: The Medieval Doctrine of Infamy'. In *Law in Medieval Life and Thought*, edited by Edward B. King, 43–89. Sewanee, TN: University of the South Press.

———. 2002. 'The Medieval Church and State on Superstition, Magic, and Witchcraft from Augustine to the Sixteenth Century'. In *Witchcraft and Magic in Europe Volume 3: The Middle Ages*. 6 vols. Edited by Bengt Ankarloo and Stuart Clark, 173–245. Philadelphia: University of Pennsylvania Press.

Pfau, Aleksandra. 2008. 'Madness in the Realm: Narratives of Mental Illness in Late Medieval France'. PhD Dissertation, University of Michigan.

———. 2010a. 'Crimes of Passion: Emotion and Madness in French Remission Letters'. In *Madness in Medieval Law and Custom*, edited by Wendy Turner, 97–122. Leiden: Brill.

———. 2010b. 'Protecting or Restraining? Madness as a Disability in Late Medieval France'. In *A World of Difference: Essays on Disability in the Middle Ages*, edited by Joshua Eyler, 93–104. London: Ashgate.

———. 2013a. 'Ritualized Violence against Sorcerers in Fifteenth-Century France'. *Magic, Ritual, and Witchcraft* Vol 8, No 1 (Summer): 50–71.

———. 2013b. 'Warfare, Trauma, and Madness in French Remission Letters'. In *The Hundred Years War (Part III): Further Considerations*, edited by L.J. Andrew Villalon and Donald J. Kagay, 437–454. Leiden: Brill.

Porter, Roy. 1987. *Mind-forg'd Manacles: A History of Madness in England from the Restoration to the Regency.* Cambridge, MA: Harvard University Press.

Pouchelle, Marie-Christine. 1990. *The Body and Surgery in the Middle Ages.* Translated by Rosemary Morris. New Brunswick, NJ: Rutgers University Press.

Presciutti, Diana Bullen. 2011. 'Dead Infants, Cruel Mothers, and Heroic Popes: The Visual Rhetoric of Foundling Care at the Hospital of Santo Spirito, Rome'. *Renaissance Quarterly* 64: 752–799.

———. 2015. *Visual Cultures of Foundling Care in Renaissance Italy.* Farnham, Surrey: Ashgate.

Prevenier, Walter. 1990. 'Violence against Women in a Medieval Metropolis: Paris Around 1400'. In *Law, Custom, and the Social Fabric in Medieval Europe: Essays in Honor of Bryce Lyon*, edited by Bernard S. Bachrach and David Nicholas, 263–284. Kalamazoo: Western Michigan University Press.

———. 1999. 'Violence against Women in Fifteenth-Century France and the Burgundian State'. In *Medieval Crime and Social Control*, edited by Barbara Hanawalt and David Wallace, 186–203. Minneapolis: University of Minnesota Press.

Puff, Helmut. 2003. *Sodomy in Reformation Germany and Switzerland, 1400–1600.* Chicago: University of Chicago Press.

Rawcliffe, Carole. 1995. *Medicine and Society in Later Medieval England*. London: Sandpiper Books.

Rider, Catherine. 2006. *Magic and Impotence in the Middle Ages*. Oxford: Oxford University Press.

Roper, Lyndal. 1994. 'Witchcraft and Fantasy in Early Modern Germany'. In *Oedipus and the Devil: Witchcraft, Sexuality and Religion in Early Modern Europe*, 199–225. London: Routledge.

———. 2004. *Witch Craze: Terror and Fantasy in Baroque Germany*. New Haven: Yale University Press.

Rorty, Richard, ed. 1967. *The Linguistic Turn: Recent Essays in Philosophical Method*. Chicago: University of Chicago Press.

Rosen, George. 1968. *Madness in Society: Chapters in the Historical Sociology of Mental Illness*. Chicago: University of Chicago Press.

Rosenthal, Joel T. 2003. *Telling Tales: Sources and Narration in Late Medieval England*. University Park: Pennsylvania State University Press.

Rosenwein, Barbara H. 2002. 'Worrying about Emotions in History'. *The American Historical Review* 107, no. 3: 821–845.

Rubin, Miri. 1987. *Charity and Community in Medieval Cambridge*. Cambridge: Cambridge University Press.

———. 1999. *Gentile Tales: The Narrative Assault on Late Medieval Jews*. New Haven: Yale University Press.

Ruggiero, Guido. 1982. 'Excusable Murder: Insanity and Reason in Early Renaissance Venice'. *Journal of Social History* 16, no. 1: 109–119.

Russell, Jeffrey Burton. 1972. *Witchcraft in the Middle Ages*. Ithaca: Cornell University Press.

Sabean, David Warren. 1984. *Power in the Blood: Popular Culture and Village Discourse in Early Modern Germany*. Cambridge: Cambridge University Press.

Salisbury, Joyce. 1994. *The Beast Within: Animals in the Middle Ages*. New York: Routledge.

Saunier, Annie. 1993. '"Hors de sens et de mémoire": une approche de la folie au travers de quelques actes judiciaires de la fin du XIIIe à la fin du XIVe siècle'. In *Commerce, finances et société (XIe–XVIe siècles): recueil de travaux d'histoire médiévale offert à M. le Professeur Henri Dubois*, edited by Philippe Contamine, Thierry Dutour, and Bertrand Schnerb, 489–500. Paris: Presses de l'Université de Paris-Sorbonne.

Saward, John. 1980. *Perfect Fools: Folly for Christ's Sake in Catholic and Orthodox Spirituality*. Oxford: Oxford University Press.

Scheff, Thomas J. 1999. *Being Mentally Ill: A Sociological Theory*. 3rd edition. New York: Aldine de Gruyter.

Schmitt, Jean-Claude. 1990. *La raison des gestes dans l'Occident médiéval*. Paris: Gallimard.

Scott, Joan. 2005. 'The Evidence of Experience'. In *Practicing History: New Directions in Historical Writing after the Linguistic Turn*, edited by Gabrielle Spiegel, 199–216. New York: Routledge.

Scull, Andrew. 1992. 'A Failure to Communicate? On the Reception of Foucault's *Histore de la folie* by Anglo-American Historians'. In *Rewriting the History of Madness: Studies in Foucault's Histoire de la folie*, edited by Arthur Still and Irving Velody, 150–163. London: Routledge.

———. 2007. 'The Fictions of Foucault's Scholarship'. *Times Literary Supplement*, March 21.

Scull, Andrew, Charlotte MacKenzie, and Nicholas Hervey. 1996. *Masters of Bedlam: The Transformation of the Mad-doctoring Trade*. Princeton: Princeton University Press.

Sigal, Pierre-André. 1985. *L'homme et le miracle dans la France médiévale (XIe–XIIe siècle)*. Paris: Les éditions du cerf.

Singer, Julie. 2018. *Representing Mental Illness in Late Medieval France: Machines, Madness, Metaphor*. Woodbridge, Suffolk: Boydell and Brewer.

Siraisi, Nancy. 1990. *Medieval and Early Renaissance Medicine: An Introduction to Knowledge and Practice*. Chicago: University of Chicago Press.

Smail, Daniel Lord. 2000. *Imaginary Cartographies: Possession and Identity in Late Medieval Marseille*. Ithaca: Cornell University Press.

———. 2003. *The Consumption of Justice: Emotions, Publicity, and Legal Culture in Marseille, 1264–1423*. Ithaca: Cornell University Press.

Soman, Alfred. 1992. *Sorcellerie et Justice Criminelle: Le Parlement de Paris (16e – 18e siècles)* Hampshire: Variorum.

Spiegel, Gabrielle. 1997. *The Past as Text: The Theory and Practice of Medieval Historiography*. Baltimore: Johns Hopkins University Press.

———, ed. 2005. *Practicing History: New Directions in Historical Writing after the Linguistic Turn*. New York: Routledge.

Steedman, Carolyn. 2002. *Dust: The Archive and Cultural History*. New Brunswick: Rutgers University Press.

Stein, Henri. 1908. *Inventaire analytique des ordonnances enregistrées au parlement de Paris jusqu'à la mort de Louis XII*. Paris: Imprimerie nationale.

Stern, Laura Ikins. 1994. *The Criminal Law System of Medieval and Renaissance Florence*. Baltimore: Johns Hopkins University Press.

Stiker, Henri-Jacques. 1999. *A History of Disability*. Translated by William Sayers. Ann Arbor: University of Michigan Press.

Stock, Brian. 1990. *Listening for the Text: On the Uses of the Past*. Baltimore: Johns Hopkins University Press.

Taylor, Craig. 2000. 'War, Propaganda and Diplomacy in Fifteenth-Century France and England'. In *War, Government and Power in Late Medieval France*, edited by Christopher Allmand, 70–91. Liverpool: Liverpool University Press.

Ternon, Maud. 2015. 'Institution judiciaire et discrédit: À propos du traitement judiciaire de la folie et de la prodigalité à la fin du Moyen Âge'. In *Faire jeunesses, rendre justice*, edited by Antoine Destemberg, Yann Potin, and Émilie Rosenblieh, 53–61. Paris: Publications de la Sorbonne.

———. 2018. *Juger les fous au Moyen Âge: Dans les tribunaux royaux en France XIVe–Xve siècles.* Paris: Presses Universitaires de France.

Texier, Pascal. 1984. 'La rémission au XIVeme siècle: Genèse et développement'. PhD dissertation, Université de Limoges.

———. 1999. 'Rémissions et ëvolutions institutionnelles'. In *Le pardon*, edited by Jacqueline Hoareau-Dodinau, Xavier Rousseaux, and Pascal Texier, 341–352. Limoges: Presses universitaires de Limoges.

———. 2001. '"Doulant et courroucié": Les avatars de la culpabilité dans les lettres de rémission du XIVème siècle'. In *La culpabilité*, edited by Jacqueline Hoareau-Dodinau and Pascal Texier, 481–494. Limoges: Presses universitaires de Limoges.

Tobler, Adolf, and Erhard Lommatzsch. 1925–. *Altfranzösisches Wörterbuch: Adolf Toblers nachgelassene Materialien bearbeitet und mit Unterstützung der Preussischen Akademie der Wissenschaften.* 11 vols. Berlin: Weidmann.

Toews, John E. 1987. 'Review: Intellectual History after the Linguistic Turn: The Autonomy of Meaning and the Irreducibility of Experience'. *The American Historical Review* 92, no. 4: 879–907.

Trenery, Claire. 2019. *Madness, Medicine and Miracle in Twelfth-century England.* London: Routledge.

Trexler, Richard C. 1981. 'La prostitution florentine au XVe siècle: Patronages et clienteles'. *Annales: Économies, sociétés, civilisations* 36, no. 6: 983–1015.

Turner, Wendy, ed. 2010. *Madness in Medieval Law and Custom*. Leiden: Brill.

———. 2013a. *Care and Custody of the Mentally Ill, Incompetent, and Disabled in Medieval England.* Turnout: Brepols.

———. 2013b. 'Defining Mental Afflictions in Medieval English Administrative Records'. In *Disability and Medieval Law: History, Literature, Society*, edited by Cory James Rushton, 134–156. Newcastle-upon-Tyne: Cambridge Scholars Publishing.

Veenstra, Jan R. 1998. *Magic and Divination at the Courts of Burgundy and France: Text and Context of Laurens Pignon's Contre les devineurs (1411).* Leiden: Brill.

Verdier, Marc. 1969. *L'église Saint-Mathurin de Larchant.* Verneuil l'Étang Amis des monuments et des sites de Seine-et-Marne.

Voegelin, Eric. 1997. *The Collected Works of Eric Voegelin Volume 21: History of Political Ideas.* Edited by David Walsh. Vol. III: The Later Middle Ages. Columbia: University of Missouri Press.

Wack, Mary Frances. 1990. *Lovesickness in the Middle Ages: The Viaticum and its Commentaries*. Philadelphia: University of Pennsylvania Press.

Walker, Nigel. 1985. 'The Insanity Defense before 1800'. *The Annals of the American Academy of Political and Social Science* 477: 25–30.

Warner, Marina. 1994. *From the Beast to the Blonde: On Fairytales and their Tellers*. London: Vintage.

Watt, Diane. 1997. 'Introduction: Medieval Women in their Communities'. In *Medieval Women in their Communities*, edited by Diane Watt, 1–19. Toronto: University of Toronto Press.

White, Hayden. 1980. 'The Value of Narrativity in the Representation of Reality'. *Critical Inquiry* 7, no. 1: 5–27.

———. 1987. *The Content of the Form: Narrative Discourse and Historical Representation*. Baltimore: Johns Hopkins University Press.

White, Stephen D. 1998. 'The Politics of Anger'. In *Anger's Past: The Social Uses of an Emotion in the Middle Ages*, edited by Barbara H. Rosenwein, 127–152. Ithaca: Cornell University Press.

Winroth, Anders. 2000. *The Making of Gratian's Decretum*. Cambridge: Cambridge University Press.

Wright, Nicholas. 1983a. 'French Peasants in the Hundred Years War'. *History Today* 33, no. 6: 38–42.

———. 1983b. '"Pillagers" and "Brigands" in the Hundred Years War'. *Journal of Medieval History* 9: 15–24.

———. 1991. 'Ransoms of Non-combatants during the Hundred Years War'. *Journal of Medieval History* 17: 323–332.

———. 1998. *Knights and Peasants: The Hundred Years War in the French Countryside*. Woodbridge, Suffolk: Boydell Press.

Wroe, Anne. 1995. *A Fool and his Money: Life in a Partitioned Medieval Town*. London: Cape.

Zink, Michel. 1976. *La prédication en langue Romane avant 1300*. Paris: Editions Honoré Champion.

Index

For Product Safety Concerns and Information please contact our EU representative GPSR@taylorandfrancis.com Taylor & Francis Verlag GmbH, Kaufingerstraße 24, 80331 München, Germany